Praise

'I commend Reena for writing this complete guide to periodontics, made possible by her knowledge of the area and, most importantly for advice on such a practical subject, her detailed experience of clinical practice. As a keystone of oral health, the periodontium is of increasing importance in our complex world, with the developing knowledge of the relationships between oral and general health. I am confident that this book will empower readers to reach professional and personal heights of excellence in the care of their patients and themselves.'
— **Dr Stephen Hancocks OBE**, former Editor-in-Chief, *BDJ*

'This is not just another book on periodontology, of which there are many. Reena has expertly captured the practical essence of the subject, and her book is packed full of down-to-earth, practical advice, analogies, hints, and tips to improve your care and communication with patients, and systems that will make delivering periodontal care rewarding, successful and always interesting.'
— **Dr Len D'Cruz**, Head of BDA Indemnity, General Dentist and Practice Owner

'Reena has dedicated her career to learning and becoming an expert in periodontics, and this handbook will be extremely useful to anyone that wants to take their perio knowledge to the next level.'
  — **Dr Yewande Oduwole**, General Dentist

'Finally! A concise, modern, and up-to-date step-by-step handbook for clinicians managing periodontics at any stage of their career.'
  — **Anna Middleton**, Dental
    Hygienist/Therapist

'As a dental student, I found this book to be an excellent resource for understanding periodontics. It's clear and easy to navigate, making it perfect for both quick reference as well as in-depth study. Covering everything from foundational knowledge to advanced surgical interventions, this book is a must-have textbook for any student looking to strengthen their knowledge in perio.'
  — **Leena Soltan**, Co-President, British Dental
    Student Association

DR REENA WADIA

THE
PERIO
HANDBOOK

THE COMPLETE GUIDE TO
MODERN PERIODONTICS

R^ethink

First published in Great Britain in 2024
by Rethink Press (www.rethinkpress.com)

Illustrations by Gemma Bull

*To my dedicated students, whose curiosity
and passion inspire me every day.*

*To the incredible team at RW Perio, for your
unwavering commitment and excellence.*

*To my talented referrers, for your trust and
collaboration in advancing periodontal care.*

*To my beloved daughter, for bringing
endless joy and perspective to my life.*

*To my wonderful husband, for your unwavering
support, encouragement, and love.*

*To my parents, for their endless sacrifices and
wisdom that have shaped who I am today.*

*And to my Guru, Pujya Mahant Swami Maharaj,
whose guidance and faith light my path.*

This book is for you all.

Contents

Foreword

The Perio Handbook, by Reena Wadia, is a refreshingly practical textbook. It delivers the complexities of periodontal and peri-implant diseases in 16 bite-sized chapters mapped into 3 parts and includes key references to ensure the contemporary evidence base is represented throughout.

Part One covers the key applied anatomy, epidemiology, pathogenesis, and risk factors across two introductory chapters.

Part Two moves onto the clinical examination process, and as well as discussing indices, looks at the initial and detailed examination process alongside clinical investigations. It covers the important area of human psychology, which is critical to gaining patient engagement, before explaining the diagnostic process by employing the British Society of Periodontology (BSP) implementation of the 2018 classification system. It finishes with concisely written sections on prognostication and peri-implant diseases.

Part Three has 10 chapters that take the reader through clinical management of periodontal and peri-implant diseases, both non-surgically and surgically. The approach employs the steps of care from the BSP's adolopment of the S3-level clinical guideline on Stages I–III periodontitis and also moves into multidisciplinary care for oral rehabilitation via orthodontic treatment, furcation management, perio–endo lesions, and periodontal emergencies. It deals with the tricky issue of palliative periodontal treatment and the importance of supportive care, focusing on real issues for patients such as recession, hypersensitivity, and halitosis. The final chapters discuss basic periodontal surgery for pocket reduction, tissue regeneration, and graft surgery.

The book successfully distils the huge evidence base of this rapidly expanding discipline into a practical guide designed for the whole dental team. It is ideal for students and new graduates, and clearly focuses on key periodontal topics for general practice.

Enjoy reading!

Professor Iain Chapple MBE

Past President of the British Society of Periodontology

Former Dean/Head of the School of Dentistry and current Director of Research for the Institute of Clinical Sciences at the University of Birmingham

European Federation of Periodontology past Treasurer, Secretary General, Founding Chair of the Scientific Affairs Committee and recipient of the 2022 Eminence Award

Introduction

Welcome to your ultimate guide to modern periodontics. This book provides a succinct yet thorough overview of the key topics that underpin the daily practice of all dental professionals. Its structure is designed to facilitate easy navigation and quick reference. The goal is to empower you with the essential knowledge and tools required to ensure the best outcomes for your patients and your practice. By following the guidelines and best practices outlined in this book, clinicians will not only enhance patient care but significantly reduce their medicolegal risk. This is particularly important given that periodontal issues are among the most common causes of dental litigation.

Part One covers the foundations, delving into the aetiology and epidemiology of periodontal diseases and providing an overview of good history taking and risk factors. Part Two looks at assessment, diagnosis, and effective patient communication strategies. Part Three explores treatment planning, providing effective oral hygiene advice in the limited time available, non-surgical periodontal therapy, and the management of specific conditions like occlusal trauma, furcations, dentine hypersensitivity, and halitosis. This section also includes protocols for managing periodontal emergencies and provides guidelines for supportive periodontal care. The final part addresses advanced topics, including the integration of dental implants in periodontitis patients, the perio–endo and perio–ortho interfaces, and various surgical interventions such as pocket reduction, gingival recession treatment, and crown-lengthening surgery. These chapters are designed to equip clinicians with the knowledge needed to handle complex cases and provide optimal patient care.

Each chapter is written with a focus on practical application, ensuring that you can easily incorporate the latest evidence-based practices into your daily routine. The book is structured to be a reliable reference, enabling you to quickly find the information you need, whether you are preparing for a procedure, educating a patient, or simply brushing up on a particular topic.

PART ONE
THE FOUNDATIONS

1
The Periodontium
And Beyond

W e begin this book by introducing its core subject matter: the periodontium. It's super important to understand the anatomy of the periodontium
in order to recognise both health and disease. We will
then outline the epidemiology and pathogenesis of
periodontitis before exploring the links between periodontitis and the rest of the body.

1.1 Anatomy of the periodontium

The periodontium's main purpose is to secure the
tooth to the jawbone and preserve the integrity of the
surface of the masticatory mucosa. Lang and Lindhe
(2015) have extensively described the anatomy of the

periodontium in their book *Clinical and Periodontology and Implant Dentistry,* but in this section we will highlight the key points.

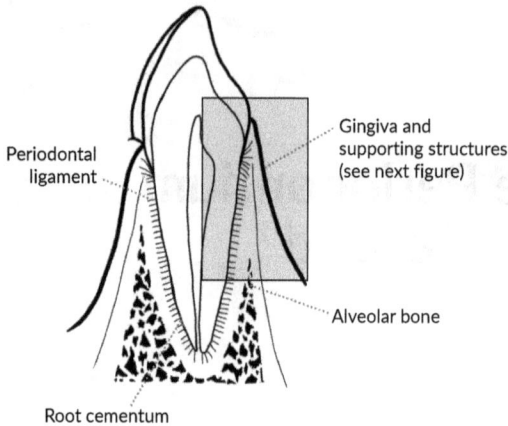

The anatomy of the periodontium in cross section

The gingiva – macroscopic

The gingivae form part of the masticatory mucosa. In the coronal direction, the gingiva terminates in the free gingival margin. In the apical direction, the gingiva is continuous with the lining mucosa, from which the gingiva is separated by the mucogingival junction. In the palate there is no mucogingival line present as the hard palate and the maxillary alveolar process are covered by the same type of masticatory mucosa.

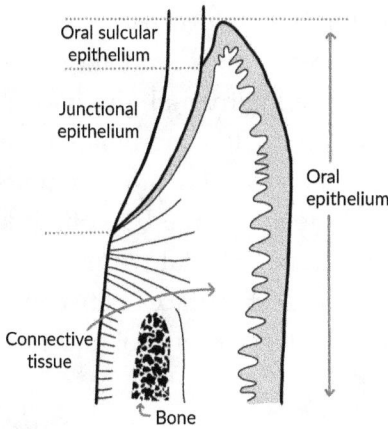

The gingiva and supporting structures in cross section

The gingiva can be divided into two regions: the free gingiva and the attached gingiva. The free gingiva, which is coral pink with a dull surface and firm consistency, includes the gingival tissue on the buccal and lingual/palatal sides of the teeth as well as the interdental papillae. It stretches from the gingival margin down to the free gingival groove, aligning with the tooth's cementoenamel junction. The attached gingiva, marked by the mucogingival junction in the apical direction, is also firm and coral pink, often exhibiting small surface indentations called 'stippling'. This part is securely attached to the underlying alveolar bone and cementum through connective tissue fibres. In contrast, the darker red alveolar mucosa below the mucogingival junction is loosely connected to the bone underneath, making it more mobile relative to the underlying tissue.

The contact points between teeth, the width of the surfaces where teeth meet, and the cementoenamel junction shape the interdental gingiva, or papilla. In the front of the mouth, the interdental papilla tends to be pyramidal, whereas in the molar regions, the papillae are more flattened in the buccolingual direction. This shape of the interdental papilla aligns with the contour of the contact surfaces between teeth, forming a concave area known as a col in the premolar and molar regions.

The gingiva – microscopic

The oral epithelium is a keratinised, stratified, squamous epithelium with distinct cell layers: the basal layer, prickle cell layer, granular cell layer, and keratinised cell layer. Besides the keratin-producing cells, which make up about 90% of the cell population, it also includes melanocytes, Langerhans cells, Merkel cells, and inflammatory cells.

The junctional epithelium has a free surface at the base of the gingival sulcus. Similar to the oral sulcular and oral epithelium, it undergoes continuous renewal via cell division in the basal layer. It narrows in the apical direction, with a thickness ranging from fifteen to thirty cells at the base of the gingival sulcus to one to three cells at its most apical end. Lacking keratinisation on its free surface, it cannot serve as a physical barrier. Hemidesmosomes and basal lamina allow the junctional epithelium cells next to the tooth to attach to its surface, while on the opposite side, these cells connect with the lamina propria of the gingiva.

The projections of connective tissue into the epithelium are known as connective tissue papillae, and are separated by epithelial ridges or rete pegs. The main tissue component of the gingiva is the connective tissue, or lamina propria. The primary components of this connective tissue are collagen fibres (60% of its volume), fibroblasts (5%), and vessels and nerves (35%), all embedded in an amorphous ground substance, or matrix. The different types of cells present in the connective tissue include fibroblasts, mast cells, macrophages, and inflammatory cells. The fibroblasts produce the connective tissue fibres, which can be classified into collagen fibres, reticulin fibres, oxytalan fibres, and elastic fibres.

The matrix of the connective tissue is primarily produced by fibroblasts, though some components are produced by mast cells, and others are derived from the blood. This matrix serves as the medium in which the connective tissue cells are embedded and is crucial for maintaining the normal function of the connective tissue. The transport of water, electrolytes, nutrients, and metabolites to and from the individual connective tissue cells takes place within this matrix. The main components of the connective tissue matrix are protein–carbohydrate macromolecules, which are typically classified into proteoglycans and glycoproteins.

Periodontal ligament

The periodontal ligament is a soft, highly vascular and cellular connective tissue that encases the roots of the teeth, linking the root cementum to the socket wall. This periodontal ligament has an hourglass shape, being narrowest at the mid-root level, and its width is about 0.25 mm (ranging from 0.2 to 0.4 mm).

The key functions of the periodontal ligament include:

- Flexible support for the teeth in their sockets (cushion)

- Sensory receptor necessary for proper positioning of the jaws

- Cell reservoir for tissue homeostasis and repair

The principal fibres of the periodontal ligament are the alveolar crest fibres, horizontal fibres, oblique fibres, and apical fibres. Sharpey's fibres are the ends of these principal fibres that are embedded in the cementum or bone, providing anchorage. The cells found in the periodontal ligament include fibroblasts (the most common cell type), osteoblasts, cementoblasts, osteoclasts, epithelial cells, and nerve fibres. As collagen matures, its fibrils contract, and there is a constant and high turnover of collagen in the periodontal ligament. This continuous process creates a permanent force that keeps the tissues firmly connected.

Root cementum

Root cementum is a specialised mineralised tissue that covers the surface of the tooth root. It connects the periodontal ligament fibres to the root and is involved in repairing any damage to the root surface.

Although root cementum shares several characteristics with bone tissue, it differs in some key aspects. Cementum lacks blood and lymph vessels, has no nerve supply, and does not undergo physiological resorption or remodelling. Instead, it continuously deposits throughout life. Like other mineralised tissues, it contains collagen fibres embedded in an organic matrix. Its mineral content, predominantly hydroxyapatite, constitutes about 65% by weight, which is slightly higher than that of bone, which is around 60%.

Alveolar bone

The alveolar bone, also known as the alveolar process, refers to the parts of the maxilla and the mandible that form and support the sockets of the teeth. The walls of the sockets are lined with cortical bone, and the area between the sockets and between the compact jawbone walls is occupied by cancellous bone. The cortical and cancellous alveolar bone are constantly undergoing remodelling (ie resorption followed by formation) with the help of osteoblasts, osteocytes, and osteoclasts.

Blood, lymphatic, and nervous supply

The dental artery, which is a branch of the superior or inferior alveolar artery, dismisses the intraseptal artery before it enters the tooth socket. The terminal branches of the intraseptal artery extend into the alveolar bone through canals at various levels within the socket. These branches form connections in the periodontal ligament space with vessels from the apical region of the periodontal ligament and other terminal branches of the intraseptal artery. Before the dental artery reaches the root canal, it gives off branches that supply the apical region of the periodontal ligament.

The gingiva's blood supply primarily comes from supraperiosteal blood vessels, which are terminal branches of the sublingual artery, mental artery, buccal artery, facial artery, greater palatine artery, infraorbital artery, and posterior superior dental artery. Lymph capillaries, which are the smallest lymph vessels, create an extensive network within the connective tissue. Like other body tissues, the periodontium contains receptors that detect pain, touch, and pressure (nociceptors and mechanoreceptors). Nerves innervate the blood vessels in the periodontium, with pain, touch, and pressure sensations having their central processing in the semilunar ganglion and travelling to the periodontium via the trigeminal nerve and its branches. The receptors in the periodontal ligament allow the detection of small forces applied to the teeth.

1.2 Periodontitis – epidemiology and pathogenesis

Periodontitis is the most prevalent chronic inflammatory disease in humans, with eight out of ten people over the age of thirty-five experiencing some form of gum issue (Chapple, 2014). Milder forms of periodontitis could affect up to 50% of individuals, while severe periodontitis impacts 11.2% of the population, making it the sixth most common health condition globally (Kassebaum et al, 2014). Despite its widespread occurrence, it remains one of the least acknowledged conditions.

Epidemiology and impact – the facts and figures

Periodontitis has been classed as a major public health problem due to its high prevalence and significant effect on quality of life. In terms of its socio-economic impact, severe periodontitis, along with dental caries, is responsible for more years lost to disability than any other human disease, and globally periodontitis is estimated to cost $54 billion in direct treatment costs and a further $25 billion in indirect costs (GBD 2017 Disease and Injury Incidence and Prevalence Collaborators, 2018). Periodontitis may also have a negative impact on general health, which will be discussed in more detail later in this chapter.

Pathogenesis

Both gingivitis and periodontitis are inflammatory conditions that occur due to the formation and persistence of microbial biofilms. Gingivitis is confined to the gingiva, while periodontitis involves additional damage to the periodontal ligament and alveolar bone. The likelihood of gingivitis advancing to periodontitis is highest among individuals who are more susceptible, accounting for approximately 5–15% of the population. In contrast, around 10% of the population appears to be resistant to periodontal damage, even with ongoing biofilm accumulation, making disease progression in these individuals uncommon (Chapple, 2014).

WHAT IS A BIOFILM?

A dental biofilm describes microorganisms attached to the tooth surface embedded in an extracellular matrix in contact with a fluid phase (Jakubovics et al, 2021). Biofilms serve as interactive microbial communities. Saliva is the primary source of nutrients for health-associated biofilms, whereas gingival crevicular fluid is a main source of nutrients for microorganisms in biofilms associated with periodontal disease.

Both the quantity and quality of bacteria that colonise the gingival sulcus can contribute to disease. These can also lead to the release of specific enzymes, toxins, and metabolic products, which have the potential for periodontal tissue damage. The bacterial flora changes with disease where more gram-negative, anaerobic, and motile bacteria, such as *Porphyromonas gingivalis*, make an appearance.

Disease occurs when there is a change in balance between the microbial biofilm and host inflammatory and immune responses. It's the host response (rather than the biofilm) that causes 80% of the tissue damage; this response is modified by local and systemic risk factors (Grossi et al, 1994). So while optimal oral hygiene remains an important factor in achieving periodontal health, it should not be the sole focus of attention. We will be discussing risk factors in more detail in Chapter 2.

Periodontitis is regarded as a condition that is seen in susceptible patients who have an exaggerated inflammatory/immune response to biofilm and/or reduced levels of defence. This leads to chronic collateral damage to the periodontal tissues because the host response is unable to successfully remove the biofilm, resulting in the propagation of the periodontal lesion. There has been debate over whether the change to the pathogenic microbial biofilm comes before or after the inflammatory response. A review by Van Dyke et al (2020) proposed that the inflammatory response is the key factor that modulates the change to the pathogenic biofilm, and it is only in the latter stages that the microbial pathogenicity becomes important.

1.3 Periodontitis and systemic disease

The whole body is connected, and the mouth should not be considered in isolation from the rest of the body. It's important to be aware of the links between periodontitis and other systemic diseases and be able to confidently discuss these with our patients. Highlighting these links can help to communicate the importance of this condition and its treatment.

The overall mechanisms linking the conditions are largely inflammatory and bacterial based. When explaining these links to patients, it's important to use them as a motivational tool rather than scaring them. Provide a positive spin on the message and use this as an opportunity to promote the importance of periodontitis prevention and treatment. Treating periodontitis and shared modifiable risk factors can only have a positive effect on related systemic disease and we dental professionals are ideally situated as front-line healthcare professionals to facilitate this.

The following are some of the systemic conditions that can be associated with periodontitis.

Diabetes

Diabetic patients with uncontrolled serum glucose levels are more likely to suffer from periodontitis compared with well-controlled diabetic or healthy individuals (Preshaw and Bissett, 2019). Periodontitis impacts the effectiveness of diabetes control and the risk of complications. Severe periodontitis affects HbA1C in individuals with and without diabetes, and moderate to severe periodontitis is associated with an increased risk of developing diabetes (Chapple et al, 2013).

Improvement of clinical periodontal parameters following standard non-surgical therapy with effective oral hygiene can be achieved even in people with poorly controlled diabetes. Randomised controlled trials consistently demonstrate that mechanical periodontal therapy is associated with a 0.4% reduction in HbA1C at three months – this impact is equivalent to adding a second drug to a pharmacological regime for diabetes (Simpson et al, 2010).

Cardiovascular disease

Periodontitis and atherosclerosis share several characteristics and mechanisms, such as the inflammatory processes and shared risk factors (age, smoking, metabolic factors, stress) as well as genetic predisposition. However, periodontitis and cardiovascular disease have been proven to be significantly associated with each other, independent of the effects of cofounders (Hirschfeld and Chapple, 2021).

Inflammatory bowel disease

Inflammatory bowel disease and periodontitis have a similar pathogenesis, characterised by a hyperactivity of the immune response to commensal microbiota in susceptible individuals (Hirschfeld and Chapple, 2021).

A meta-analysis of nine observational studies from different populations reported a 4.5-fold higher periodontitis risk in adult patients with inflammatory bowel disease. The overall quality of evidence should be considered weak-moderate; however, the existing studies report a significant association (Hirschfeld and Chapple, 2021).

Rheumatoid arthritis

There appears to be a clear epidemiological relationship between rheumatoid arthritis and periodontitis, although the directionality of this relationship is not known. Based on the current evidence, a causal relationship cannot be proven, and, if proven in the future, it may be an association in a subset of susceptible rheumatoid arthritis patients only (Hirschfeld and Chapple, 2021). Future research is needed to investigate this.

Respiratory diseases

While there are plausible mechanisms explaining the potential associations between periodontitis and several respiratory diseases, a lack of epidemiological evidence means associations in general are inconclusive (Hirschfeld and Chapple, 2021).

Adverse pregnancy outcomes and fertility

There appears to be a modest association between periodontitis and pre-eclampsia and weak evidence of an association between periodontal diseases and pre-term and low-birth weight. Both associations are hampered by the heterogeneity of the data. Despite extensive research spanning over twenty-five years, definitive conclusions about the relationships between periodontal health and negative pregnancy outcomes remain elusive (Hirschfeld and Chapple, 2021).

Pregnancy can impact periodontal health due to changes in sex hormone levels, which may increase gingival inflammation. This effect is likely linked to the presence of oral biofilms, increased blood flow and vascularity, and cellular alterations. Additionally, these hormonal changes can heighten the inflammatory response to the biofilm, potentially leading to oedematous changes or the development of a localised area of highly vascular granulation tissue, known as an epulis.

Regarding fertility, there is extremely limited and weak evidence that periodontal disease is associated with infertility. Larger observational studies that adjust for confounding factors need to be implemented (Hirschfeld and Chapple, 2021).

Neurodegenerative diseases

Knowledge in this field is still in its infancy, but it is known that the progression of cognitive decline has a marked effect on individual dental biofilm control (Hirschfeld and Chapple, 2021).

There is an indication that for a proportion of those who develop the common non-familial Alzheimer's disease, periodontitis could be involved in the progression, if not the initiation of their condition. There is clear epidemiological evidence of an association between the two conditions of periodontitis and Alzheimer's disease, which are both pro-inflammatory. Furthermore, there is evidence that the co-existence of periodontitis is associated with more rapid rates of cognitive decline, suggesting that the presence of periodontitis has an adverse effect on the progression of Alzheimer's disease (Hirschfeld and Chapple, 2021).

The evidence for a link between periodontitis and Parkinson's disease is largely circumstantial. However, this is likely to become clearer with more studies. Overall, further evidence is required to determine whether any causative association between periodontitis and neurodegenerative disease exists.

Stress and depression

Both stress and depression dysregulate the immune response and produce changes in the central and peripheral nervous and endocrine systems. Psychological factors can change health-related behaviour, leading to unhealthy habits including alcohol and substance abuse, cigarette smoking, and neglect of oral hygiene. These factors contribute to a higher risk of periodontitis (Hirschfeld and Chapple, 2021).

2
Think Like A Detective

When dealing with patients with periodontitis, it's important to think like a detective. Every patient sitting in your chair has a 'causal pie' above their head and although biofilm/suboptimal oral hygiene will be a slice of that pie, you need to find out what the rest of the slices are. These will be different for every patient and, if they are not identified, the accuracy of the diagnosis and success of the treatment plan will be affected.

You need to think like a detective when it comes to working out whether and why the patient has periodontitis. In the first instance, identifying a periodontitis patient requires thorough history taking, which relies on asking the right questions. Then, when trying to figure out the cause, a consideration of risk factors comes into play.

2.1 History taking – asking the right questions

There are four quick trigger questions to ask all patients. If they answer yes to any of these, this is a clue that they may be a periodontitis patient:

1. **Do your gums bleed on brushing?** It's important to include 'on brushing' as often patients will think it's normal that their gums bleed on brushing so may answer no if you ask them only if their gums bleed. If they say no to this, then you can question them about bleeding when using floss or interdental brushes.

2. **Are any of your teeth loose?** Loose teeth are a strong indicator of periodontitis. You can also ask them if the looseness is affecting their ability to eat comfortably.

3. **Any gum swellings or gum boils?** Often patients won't understand what an abscess is so using the term 'gum boil' is helpful.

4. **Do you suffer from bad breath or notice a bad taste?** Individuals might be embarrassed to admit to bad breath, but tend to be happier to admit to a bad taste, so always lead with this.

As well as serving as diagnostic clues, the above trigger questions might reveal the patient's 'pain point' – the reason they are seeking treatment. Being aware of this means we can discuss how we will address it through treatment, increasing motivation for treatment uptake and aiding patient compliance.

2.2 Systemic risk factors

A risk factor is an occurrence or characteristic associated with the increased rate of a subsequently occurring disease (Van Dyke and Dave, 2005). The presence of biofilm is like the key having been turned in a car's ignition, but all the other risk factors are pressing on the accelerator, driving the disease forward. Systemic risk factors may be among the key determinants of susceptibility. Risk factors may affect the periodontal tissues, host response, or the oral environment. They may be modifiable or non-modifiable. They might also influence the treatment approach, so you must ensure you pick up the key risk factors for periodontitis during your history taking.

When you take your patient's history, go through this in a logical order, addressing the medical history, social history, and dental history, all of which are relevant to periodontal disease.

Medical history

When taking the patient's medical history, there are several key risk factors to watch out for, notably diabetes, pregnancy, immunodeficiency and any medications the patient may be taking.

Diabetes

Diabetes is a group of metabolic disorders characterised by hyperglycaemia resulting from the body's inability to control blood glucose (lack of insulin/responsiveness). According to the International Diabetes Federation, diabetes is now a global epidemic with 50% of cases being undiagnosed (IDF, 2021). There are three main types: type 1, type 2, and gestational.

Patients with hyperglycaemia are three times more likely to develop periodontitis (Chapple and Genco, 2013).

Diabetes increases patients' susceptibility to and the severity of periodontitis. It is classed as a modifiable risk factor as, though it cannot be cured, it can be controlled, and control is the most important factor related to this condition.

Practical tips for dealing with periodontitis patients with diabetes:

- Ensure your patient has eaten before any treatment appointments to minimise risk of a hypoglycaemic episode.

- Check the patient's glycaemic control by asking for the results of a recent HbA1C test or by completing one on-site. The HbA1C level (which is a measure of three-month control) should ideally be <6.5% / 48 mmol / mol.

- Poorly controlled diabetics will be at higher risk of periodontitis so may require more frequent periodontal examinations.

- Poor glycaemic control reduces the benefits of periodontal therapy. Ensure the patient is aware of this and make a note of the fact you have emphasised the importance of good control.

- Be a supporter when it comes to oral hygiene. Diabetics have many other general health issues to worry about so try and see how you can fit oral hygiene into their overall self-care regime.

- Following successful periodontal treatment, HbA1C reductions of 0.4% have been shown – a clinical equivalent to adding a second drug to a pharmacological regime for diabetes (Chapple et al, 2013). This can be hugely motivational for patients.

Pregnancy

Stimulation of prostaglandin synthesis can result in vascular changes. Hormonal changes mean that the inflammatory effects are magnified if the dental biofilm is not adequately controlled; this results in oedematous and/or proliferative alterations. The classic proliferative change is a pregnancy epulis.

Practical tips for working with pregnant patients, as suggested by the European Federation of Periodontology:

- Identify the stage of pregnancy and perform a comprehensive periodontal examination.

- Pregnant women with a healthy periodontium should be provided with oral health education, including detailed oral hygiene instructions.

- Emphasise to patients with gingivitis or periodontitis that non-surgical periodontal therapy during pregnancy is safe, effective, and beneficial.

- Following treatment, reassess the periodontal status according to normal practice.

- Once treated, frequent monitoring of the periodontal condition should be maintained throughout pregnancy and if there is a recurrence, a similar intervention should be provided.

- For a pregnancy epulis, surgical excision can be performed for large lesions that are impacting upon function or aesthetics. However, if lesions are small, excision can be delayed until postpartum with supportive measures carried out during pregnancy.

- If possible, other forms of elective periodontal surgery should also be avoided during pregnancy.

It's also important to be aware of other hormonal changes, as they will impact on periodontitis risk; this includes puberty and the menopause.

Immunodeficiency

Ensure you closely examine immunodeficient patients as they can present with necrotising periodontal disease (necrotising gingivitis or periodontitis). Signs of necrotising disease include a pseudomembrane, punched-out papillae, and halitosis. Immunodeficiency can be the result of HIV/AIDS but in this case the signs may be subtle, as medications can now control HIV/AIDS very well.

Necrotising periodontal disease is also not uncommon in patients with high stress levels, those who are run down, smokers, and those with suboptimal oral hygiene. Treatment includes gentle professional mechanical plaque removal, adjunctive use of a mouthwash, and metronidazole antibiotics.

Medications

The role of biofilm in the overall pathogenesis is now regarded as important, with most studies indicating that biofilm is a prerequisite for gingival enlargement to occur. The gingival enlargement then makes it more difficult to maintain optimal plaque control (Zoheir and Hughes, 2020). There are certain medications that increase the risk of gingival enlargement in certain individuals (Zoheir and Hughes, 2020). Look out for phenytoin (anticonvulsant for epilepsy), cyclosporin (immunosuppressive for transplant patients), and -dipine medications, for example amlodipine (calcium-channel blocker for hypertension).

FACTS ABOUT DRUG-INFLUENCED GINGIVAL ENLARGEMENT

- The first signs of change are reported to arise about one to three months following the start of dosing.
- There appears to be a minimum threshold for drug plasma levels, below which drug-influenced gingival enlargement is unlikely to occur.
- Phenytoin causes a largely fibrotic and pink enlargement, whereas calcium-channel blockers are associated with a more vascular overgrowth.
- Enlargement classically begins at the interdental papilla region.

Practical tips on managing patients with gingival enlargement as a result of prescribed medication:

- Ensure you have an up-to-date medical history.

- Contact the patient's general medical practitioner (GMP) to find out if it would be feasible to replace the risk factor drug with an alternative. This might occur following initial therapy or at the start if the overgrowth is severe.

- Oral hygiene reinforcement, with an emphasis on angulation into the gingival sulcus area, is particularly helpful here. Single-tufted brushes are a useful adjunct.

- Complete a Basic Periodontal Examination (BPE) and six-point pocket chart if needed. Radiographic examination will be key to work out if there are areas of false pocketing.

- Carry out supragingival and subgingival professional mechanical plaque removal as necessary. Ensure that any plaque-retentive factors, such as overhanging restorations, have been corrected.

- Surgery may be indicated following non-surgical therapy if the enlarged tissues are significant and very fibrous.

- Regular supportive periodontal therapy will be key to minimise recurrence.

Below is an example letter to a GMP, which can be used to request the exploration of an alternative drug if required.

Dear Dr [Name]

Re: [Name, address, DOB]

I recently saw this patient regarding his gum issues.

I understand he is a patient of yours who is hypertensive and taking [insert drug and dose].

On examination today, there was significant gum swelling/enlargement, and he has been diagnosed with [insert detailed periodontitis diagnosis]. This condition is having a significant impact on his daily quality of life.

As you will know, calcium channel blockers are well recognised to sometimes have adverse effects on the gums, and his condition is typical of calcium-channel blocker-associated periodontal disease.

I am writing to ask if you would be able to assess him to consider whether it may be possible for you to change his medication to a non-calcium channel blocker antihypertensive drug?

Best wishes,

Dr [Name]

[You can also include photos to emphasise the impact]

Family history/genetics

Interestingly, 50% of periodontitis susceptibility is due to host genetic factors (Michalowicz et al, 2000). Evidence for this association is stronger for Grade C forms of periodontitis, where the attachment loss can be inconsistent with local risk factors. It may be helpful in these cases to tell patients that 'periodontitis can be an unfair condition.' Patients may often mention a family history of periodontitis, but the reliability can vary; for example, if a patient says that their thirty-two-year-old sibling is having surgery for periodontitis, that is likely more reliable than someone mentioning that their parents had weak gums and lost all their teeth early.

Social history

As well as medical and family history, it's also important to look at the patient's social history, to identify further potential risk factors, including the following.

Smoking

While the prevalence of smoking has decreased steadily across the globe, it remains a common risk factor for periodontitis. In fact, 42% of periodontitis may be attributable to smoking (Tomar and Asma, 2000). Smoking increases susceptibility to and severity of periodontitis in a dose-dependent manner.

Smokers will have deeper pockets, more recession, greater bone loss (especially in the upper anterior regions), and increased tooth loss compared to non-smokers (Tomar and Asma, 2000). Smokers are likely to also have less marginal bleeding, masking the early critical signs of periodontitis (Bergstrom and Bostrom, 2001).

Local effects of smoking include reduced tissue vascularity, as well as impaired polymorphonuclear leucocyte chemotaxis and function. Systemic effects include decreased salivary IgA, decreased serum IgG, and decreased helper T cells (Ryder et al, 1998).

For smokers, there will be poorer success rates in both non-surgical and surgical therapy with a greater chance of disease recurrence (Ah et al, 1994; Bostrom et al, 1998). During maintenance, smokers will be more likely to lose teeth than non-smokers. This all needs to be discussed with the patient and clearly noted in their records.

Some practical tips on facilitating smoking cessation:

- Don't underestimate the impact of your role, even if it's a brief intervention (Ramseier et al, 2020). Smoking cessation is essential. **Ask** (them if they are interested in stopping), **advise** (them on the benefits for both general and oral health), and **refer** (to smoking cessation services, if they are keen).

- Use of NHS stop-smoking services (nhs.uk/ smokefree) almost triples the likelihood of successfully quitting.

- Focus on the advantages of quitting rather than the disadvantages of not quitting.

Vaping

Research shows that 37% of current smokers vape, so it's important to ask them about this (ASH, 2023). Vaping is reportedly better for general health and is an effective tool to help smokers quit. The effects of vaping on the periodontal condition are unknown, but most professionals speculate that nicotine will likely have some negative impact, so in the long-term, vaping cessation should be a part of the treatment plan (Holliday et al, 2021).

Stress

Stress is a significant risk factor for periodontitis, especially when there is evidence of poor coping strategies (Wimmer et al, 2002; Hugoson, Ljungquist, and Breivik, 2002). Ask patients about their stress levels and negative life events. The mechanisms underlying this association are not well understood but include a mix of behavioural changes and impact on the immune system.

Dental history

Of course, the patient's dental history is relevant to a diagnosis and assessment of periodontitis, and history taking in this regard should cover the following.

Diet/nutrition

Nutrition will modify the severity and extent of the disease by affecting host resistance and potential for repair, and some nutritional deficiencies may exacerbate gingival response to plaque (Raindi, 2016). For example, micronutrient deficiencies have been shown to be inversely related to periodontal health. Specifically, there is good quality evidence for an association with vitamin C, magnesium/calcium levels, antioxidants, docosahexaenoic acid, and vitamin D (Woelber et al, 2017). At a macronutrient level, emerging evidence indicates that a carbohydrate-rich diet increases the risk of inflammation and, thus, gingival bleeding, whereas a switch to a palaeolithic diet results in a decrease in gingival bleeding (Raindi, 2016).

When talking to patients about diet and nutrition, ensure that you:

- Explain the potential dietary impact on both systemic and oral disease

- Encourage a well-balanced diet

- Explain that diet modification is preferred over the use of supplements

2.3 Local risk factors

Successful treatment will be dependent on detailed history-taking to pick up the above risk factors, as these require appropriate management. When examining the patient, further local risk factors may also be noted. These act as biofilm-retentive factors, increasing the risk of periodontitis. Examples include:

- Calculus

- Root caries and severe abrasive tooth wear

- Restorations – overhangs, open margins

- Orthodontic appliances, dentures, and crown/bridge work if not of a hygienic design

- Anatomical, eg enamel pearls or root grooves

- Crowded dentition

- High frenal attachment

- Mouth breathing/incompetent lip seal/xerostomia

During the treatment of periodontitis, we need to tackle systemic patient-level, mouth-level, tooth-level, and, finally, site-level risk factors.

PART TWO
ASSESSMENT AND DIAGNOSIS

3
Clinical Examination

Before a treatment plan can be designed, a thorough clinical examination must take place. During the examination it's important to assess the appearance of the gingivae as well as the level of biofilm control. Probing is imperative when assessing the periodontium and comfortable probing is a must-have skill. As part of the clinical assessment, one should also be confident in assessing dental implants.

3.1 Appearance of the gingivae

Before probing, there must be a visual assessment of the gingivae during which the following three categories should be considered:

1. **Colour:** Healthy gingivae are typically described as 'coral pink' and will be paler in colour than inflamed gingivae, which may appear redder in colour.

2. **Contour:** A healthy gingiva will have a scalloped shape, tightly adapted to the underlying tissues, and a knife-edge margin where it abuts the tooth.

3. **Consistency:** Inflamed gingivae will appear swollen and 'spongy' in texture.

Make a note of the gingival phenotype. It would be considered thin if you can see the probe shining through the gingival sulcus when probing, and thick if not. Teeth tend to be more triangular shaped in thin phenotypes and squarer in thick.

3.2 Assessment of biofilm

A general subjective assessment of biofilm/plaque control is often completed, but objective measurements through scores are more useful. Several systems for scoring biofilm exist. Two common examples are the Simplified Plaque Index by Ainamo and Bay (1975) and the Plaque Control Record developed by O'Leary et al (1972).

The Simplified Plaque Index (Ainamo and Bay, 1975)

This index consists of two possible scores:

- 0 – no plaque detected
- 1 – visible plaque detected

This dichotomous system makes a note of whether there is plaque detected or no plaque detected for each tooth. This can then be used to produce a percentage score.

The Plaque Control Record (O'Leary et al, 1972)

This system was developed to provide a simple method of recording the presence of biofilm/plaque on individual tooth surfaces – ie mesial, distal, buccal, and lingual/palatal. The teeth are disclosed, and each surface of the tooth is examined. Those with plaque are recorded. After all the teeth have been examined, the index is calculated by dividing the number of plaque-containing surfaces by the total number of available surfaces, and this is expressed as a percentage.

One disadvantage of the plaque score is that it gives only a snapshot of the patient's oral hygiene compliance at that moment in time. Marginal bleeding may be a more reliable measure of the patient's ability to remove accessible plaque and control marginal inflammation.

Marginal bleeding is different to bleeding on probing. For marginal bleeding the probe is run only along the gingival margin and for bleeding on probing you probe to the base of the pocket.

The Simplified Gingival Index (Ainamo and Bay, 1975)

As a supplement to plaque measurement instruments, the Simplified Gingival Index from Ainamo and Bay (1975) is a commonly used gingival index for marginal bleeding, with scores as follows:

- 0 – no bleeding from the gingival margin detected after a periodontal probe is briefly run along the gingival margin
- 1 – bleeding from the gingival margin detected after a periodontal probe is briefly run along the gingival margin

While assessing biofilm, it is helpful to also assess calculus. This can be completed through a visual assessment with a note made of the presence or absence of supragingival and/or subgingival calculus.

3.3 Making probing comfortable

Ensure your probing is as comfortable as possible for the patient. For them, this will be a preview of your future care; if they have an unpleasant experience, this may affect their acceptance of the treatment plan. There are both communication and technique tips to help with this.

Communication tips for probing:

1. **Explain and prewarn:** Prior to probing, explain to the patient that you will be completing 'gum measurements, which are the only way to check the health of the gums.' This ensures they fully understand why you need to probe. They should also be aware that if their gums are inflamed, the probing may be slightly uncomfortable, but give them the option of raising their hand to ask you to stop if they need a breather. If there is some discomfort, rather than the patient thinking you are causing the pain, their main concern should be the fact they may have gum disease. By explaining and pre-warning there is a mindset shift from the start.

2. **Praise:** It is not the most pleasant experience for our patients so praising them on how well they are doing as you are probing can be helpful. Also let them know when you are more than halfway through, especially when completing full pocket charts.

3. **Conversation after:** If specific areas were sore, use this to your advantage and explain why they might have been more uncomfortable. This will engage the patient and link in well when explaining the aetiology and treatment of gum disease.

Technique tips for probing:

- **Sweep/drag the probe:** Don't keep taking the probe in and out of the pocket, potentially 'stabbing' the patient 192 times.

- **Appropriate pressure:** Let the probe drop into the pocket (no additional pressure) – technically you are aiming for 25 g, the amount of force necessary to just blanch your fingernail when pushing on it.

- **Finger rest:** Use a finger rest, as close as possible to the tooth being probed, to ensure good pressure control.

- **Appropriate angulation:** Angle the probe along the root surface.

- **Topical anaesthesia:** Oraqix (lidocaine and prilocaine gel) may be helpful in certain cases.

- **Recheck probing once numbed up for treatment:** If the patient is extremely uncomfortable, recheck the probing depths once anaesthetised for treatment and adjust if needed.

- **Good vision:** Using loupes with a light will provide good vision to ensure you're not having to repeatedly probe to recheck measurements.

3.4 The BPE

The Basic Periodontal Examination (BPE) (2019) is the primary and minimum standard of care for periodontal assessment in the UK. It's a rapid screening tool that indicates when further examination is required and suggests basic guidance on the treatment needed.

The BPE consists of three steps, as follows:

1. Ensure you are using a BPE (WHO) probe – this has a 'ball end' 0.5 mm in diameter and a black band from 3.5–5.5 mm.

2. Divide the dentition into six sextants and record the highest score for each sextant. For a sextant to qualify for recording, it must contain at least two teeth.

3. Probe all teeth in each sextant (except for the third molars unless the first and/or second molars are missing). Even if a Code 4 is identified in a sextant, you should continue to examine all sites in the sextant.

Scoring codes summary

0	Probing depth < 3.5 mm	Black band entirely visible. No calculus/ overhangs, no bleeding on probing.	No need for periodontal treatment. Record BPE at every routine examination.
1	Pockets depth < 3.5 mm	Black band entirely visible. No calculus/ overhangs, bleeding on probing.	Oral hygiene instruction. Record BPE at every routine examination.
2	Pockets depth < 3.5 mm	Black band entirely visible. Supra or subgingival calculus/ overhangs.	As for Code 1, plus removal of plaque-retentive factors, including all supra and subgingival calculus. Record BPE at every routine examination.
3	Probing depth 3.5– 5.5 mm	Black band partially visible.	Initial therapy including self-care advice (oral hygiene instruction and risk factor control) then, post-initial therapy, record a six-point pocket chart in that sextant only. Ensure appropriate radiographs are available.
4	Probing depth > 5.5 mm	Black band disappears.	Record a six-point pocket chart throughout the entire dentition then treatment plan. Assess the need for more complex treatment; referral to a specialist may be indicated. Ensure appropriate radiographs are available.

*	Furcation involvement	Both the above code and a * should be recorded if furcation involvement is detected.	Treat according to BPE Codes 0–4. Assess the need for more complex treatment; referral to a specialist may be indicated.

Example BPE score

3	2	3*
4	2	-

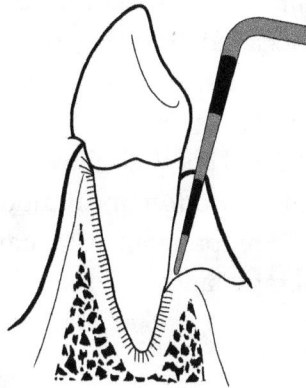

Probing showing a BPE score of 4

If the patient is under the age of eighteen, a simplified BPE should be performed. This involves assessing six index teeth (UR6, UR1, UL6, LL6, LL1, and LR6). BPE Codes 0–2 are used in seven to eleven-year-olds, while the full range of codes (0, 1, 2, 3, 4, and *) can be used in twelve to seventeen-year-olds.

3.5 The six-point pocket chart

Remember, the BPE cannot be used to monitor the response to periodontal therapy because it does not provide information about how sites within a sextant change after treatment; it is just a screening tool. To assess the response to treatment, a six-point pocket chart should be completed pre- and post-treatment.

A full pocket chart involves taking measurements at six sites per tooth – mesial, mid, distal on both the buccal and palatal/lingual aspects. Periodontal probing depths, associated bleeding on probing (BoP), and gingival recession will be measured. Mobility and furcation involvement will also be noted on a full pocket chart. This will allow a more detailed assessment of the periodontal condition to aid treatment planning. For patients who have undergone periodontal therapy and are receiving supportive periodontal care, a full pocket chart is recommended at least annually.

The probing depth is the distance from the gingival margin to the location of the tip of the periodontal probe. This may or may not be the true histological attachment loss and, hence, the term probing depth is more appropriate than pocket depth. According to the British Society of Periodontology's (BSP) (2019) guidance, when a six-point pocket chart is indicated it is only necessary to record sites of 4 mm and above (although six sites per tooth should be measured).

BoP is the most important measure of current periodontal disease status and should always be recorded. It refers to the presence or absence of bleeding following probing to the base of the pocket, where BoP indicates the presence of inflammation. If there is suppuration (pus), this can also be noted.

Recession is the distance from the cementoenamel junction to the gingival margin. Identifying the exact level of the cementoenamel junction can be tricky and may often need to be estimated.

Probing depth + recession = clinical attachment loss

To measure mobility, use the other side of your probe and mirror handle and apply light force, alternating first one way and then the other. Observe the tooth for movement buccolingually/mesiodistally as well as vertically. The most commonly used system to record mobility was created by Miller (1950).

Miller's (1950) measure of mobility

0	Physiological mobility (0.1–0.2 mm in horizontal direction)
1	0.2–1 mm horizontal movement
2	1–2 mm horizontal movement
3	Excess of 2 mm horizontal movement or any vertical movement

Furcation involvement is usually assessed with probing, but radiographs can also help with interpretation.

A curved Nabers probe can be used if needed. Each furcation entrance must be classified separately. There are several classification systems; a commonly used one is that by Hamp et al (1975).

Hamp et al's (1975) furcation classification system

I	Loss of horizontal periodontal support not exceeding one-third of the width of the tooth
II	Loss of horizontal probing support exceeding one-third of the width of the tooth but not encompassing the total width of the furcation
III	'Through-and-through' destruction of periodontal tissues in the furcation area

3.6 Assessment of dental implants

Assess the colour, contour, and consistency of the peri-implant tissues as well as the oral hygiene. The BPE should not be used around implants; instead, complete a four- or six-point pocket chart. Routine gentle probing using your standard (metal) probe is safe. Make a note of the absence or presence of any bleeding or suppuration on probing.

4

Special Investigations

The next step in the assessment journey after the clinical examination and prior to making any diagnoses, is the special investigation phase.

4.1 Radiographs

Radiographs are the key method to assess bone levels. The type of radiograph required is a matter of clinical judgement and this decision should also take into consideration the overall dental needs of the patient. For periodontal assessment, ensure the crestal bone levels are visible in all areas. For mild bone loss, this may be captured through standard horizontal bitewing radiographs. For more extensive disease, many clinicians would regard periapical radiographs as essential to allow accurate assessment of bone loss as a percentage of root length and visualisation of periapical tissues. Dental panoramic radiographs can be helpful if there are other issues, for example impacted third molars, or if orthodontic assessment is needed, but supplemental periapical radiographs may be required anteriorly, as bone levels are often not shown as clearly here due to the superimposition of the spine.

The clinical need will determine the frequency of radiographic exposure required. Before taking updated radiographs, always ask yourself, 'Will this change how I treat the patient?' If it will not, you should question why the radiograph is being taken.

Once you have assessed whether the radiographs are diagnostic or not, report on the following five features:

1. **Amount of bone loss** – in millimetres or, if you can see the root apex, then percentage

2. **Pattern of bone loss** – horizontal or vertical

3. **Local factors** – check for any evidence of calculus, restorative overhangs, or open margins

4. **Anatomy** – root length and morphology. Do not underestimate the importance of assessing this, as it will have a significant impact on the prognosis of a tooth

5. **Widening** of the periodontal ligament space and signs of any periapical pathology

When reading radiographs, scan in the same direction every time – coronal to apical, or apical to coronal – this ensures you do not miss any important details.

4.2 Sensibility testing

Sensibility testing assesses sensory/nerve supply to the tooth. If this is negative, it may highlight any endo–perio lesions in more extensive disease.

Sensibility testing can be completed via thermal tests, such as Endo-Frost, or through electric tests – eg an electric pulp tester can be used to indirectly determine the state of pulpal health by assessing the condition of the nerves within the dental pulp. Although false positives and negatives may be encountered, these tests can be helpful in identifying endo–perio lesions.

5
Diagnosis

I t's now time to bring all the information together to come up with a periodontal diagnosis or diagnoses. Formulating a diagnosis is imperative prior to prescribing a treatment plan for the patient. We will explore the updated classification and discuss periodontal health, gingival diseases, periodontitis, other conditions of the periodontium and peri-implant disease.

5.1 Background

The 2017 World Workshop introduced a new classification system for periodontal and peri-implant diseases and conditions, reflecting significant advancements in biological and clinical research since the 1999

International Classification of Periodontal Diseases (Caton et al, 2018). This revised system now explicitly defines clinical health and differentiates between an intact and a reduced periodontium. It has eliminated the terms 'aggressive' and 'chronic' periodontitis, replacing them with a staging and grading framework for periodontitis. To facilitate the application of this updated classification in UK clinical settings, the BSP established an implementation group to provide relevant guidance (Dietrich et al, 2019).

5.2 Periodontal health and gingival diseases

The first part of the updated classification focuses on periodontal health and gingival diseases.

Periodontal health

Pristine periodontal health is very rare. 'Clinical health' has been defined as probing depths of 3 mm or below, as well as less than 10% bleeding on probing (Chapple et al, 2018).

Clinical gingival health may occur on an intact periodontium – in other words, in the absence of detectable attachment and/or bone loss – or on a reduced periodontium, either in a stable periodontitis patient or non-periodontitis patient (Chapple et al, 2018).

Gingivitis: Dental biofilm-induced

Gingivitis that is dental biofilm-induced is defined as an inflammatory lesion resulting from interactions between the biofilm and the host's immune-inflammatory response. It remains confined to the gingiva and is reversible. A diagnosis of gingivitis can be made if 10% or more of sites exhibit bleeding on probing (Chapple et al, 2018).

Gingivitis can develop on an intact periodontium or on a reduced periodontium in an individual who has not had periodontitis. Additionally, gingival inflammation might occur on a reduced periodontium in a patient who has been successfully treated for periodontitis.

Gingivitis: Non-dental biofilm-induced

This form of gingivitis is not triggered by biofilm and typically does not improve after biofilm removal. Non-dental biofilm-induced gingivitis may present as part of a systemic condition or be localised to the oral cavity. A key distinction from dental biofilm-induced gingivitis is that the inflammation here extends beyond the mucogingival junction, while in biofilm-related gingivitis the inflammation will remain more localised.

These are categorised under: a) genetic/developmental; b) specific infections; c) inflammatory/immune;

d) reactive; e) neoplasms; f) endocrine, nutritional and metabolic; g) traumatic; h) pigmentation (Chapple et al, 2018).

5.3 Periodontitis

There are now only three types of periodontitis: necrotising periodontal diseases, periodontitis, and periodontitis as a manifestation of systemic disease (Dietrich et al, 2019). Let's start off with periodontitis, as this is the type that will be seen most often in practice and that clinicians need to be super confident in diagnosing.

Periodontitis

The most efficient way of coming up with the diagnostic statement for periodontitis patients is by following the below six steps:

1. **Periodontitis:** The first step is to determine if they are a periodontitis patient by reviewing the available radiographs and checking for any bone loss. If there is bone loss due to periodontitis, then they will be labelled as a 'periodontitis' patient regardless of their clinical status. This is key as, once a patient is diagnosed as such, they are a periodontitis patient for life – they need to know this to ensure they keep up supportive periodontal care. Be aware that bone loss can

happen due to other reasons, such as surgical extractions, crown-lengthening procedures, or other pathology.

2. **Extent:** Assess the radiographs to determine the extent of bone loss. This can be divided into:

   - Localised: up to 30% of teeth with bone loss

   - Generalised: more than 30% of teeth with bone loss

   - Molar–incisor pattern: first molars with/ without incisors affected

3. **Stage:** The stage refers to the severity of the disease and can be assessed as a percentage of the root length on periapical/dental panoramic radiographs, or estimated from bitewings. Pick the tooth with the most interproximal bone loss and classify as follows:

   - Stage I (early/mild) – less than 15% bone loss or less than 2 mm (measurement from cementoenamel junction (CEJ) if only bitewings available)

   - Stage II (moderate) – coronal third of root

   - Stage III (severe) – mid-third of root

   - Stage IV (very severe) – apical third of root

Note: In situations where it is clear that a patient has lost teeth due to advanced periodontal bone loss, likely within the apical third of the root, you may, on a case-by-case basis, immediately classify this as Stage IV.

4. **Grade:** The grading is designed to reflect the patient's susceptibility to periodontitis and provides a good predictor of future disease experience in the absence of treatment. The quickest way of grading a patient is to apply the following:

   - Grade A is assigned if the greatest amount of radiographic bone loss, in percentage terms, is less than half the patient's age in years.

   - Grade C is assigned if the greatest amount of bone loss, in percentage terms, exceeds the patient's age in years.

   - Grade B is assigned otherwise.

5. **Current disease status:** So far, the focus has been on bone levels. This next step is about understanding what we will be treating / maintaining by determining the patient's disease status. The patient may be:

   - Stable – healthy / successfully treated

   - Disease remission – bleeding on probing more than or equal to 10% of sites, with probing depths of less than or equal to 3 mm and no probing depths of greater than 4 mm

   - Unstable – bleeding sites in probing depths of 4 mm or more or any probing depth of 5 mm and above

6. **Risk factor profile:** The final step includes making a note of whether the patient is diabetic and/or a (previous) smoker. These risk factors form part of the diagnostic statement as they can be measured and controlled. Any other risk factors can be noted on a separate line from the diagnostic statement, as these are still important to acknowledge to ensure we have a full picture of the patient's 'causal pie'.

Necrotising periodontal diseases

These diseases rank among the most severe inflammatory conditions associated with dental biofilm. They include necrotising gingivitis and necrotising periodontitis. Necrotising gingivitis is limited to the gum tissues, and necrotising periodontitis is where the necrosis extends into the periodontal ligament and alveolar bone, causing attachment loss (Papapanou et al, 2018). The mandibular anterior teeth are the most frequently affected.

Necrotising gingivitis is marked by necrosis and ulceration in the free gingiva. These lesions typically begin at the interdental papilla and often have the classic 'punched-out' appearance. Marginal erythema may be seen, and the necrotic lesions can extend to the marginal gingiva. A pseudo-membrane may cover the necrotic area; removing this 'membrane' exposes the underlying connective tissue, which then bleeds. The level of pain experienced by the patient varies depending on the severity and extent of the lesions, typically intensifying during eating and oral hygiene activities. Less common symptoms include halitosis, fever, and malaise.

Necrotising periodontitis shares the features of necrotising gingivitis but additionally involves necrosis of the periodontal ligament and alveolar bone, leading to attachment loss. As the disease advances, an interproximal crater forms, separating the buccal and lingual/palatal portions of the papilla. If these craters deepen, the interdental crestal bone can become exposed. When interproximal necrotic areas extend laterally and merge, they create a large zone of tissue destruction. In severe cases, bone sequestration may occur. Risk factors include high stress levels, heavy smoking, and poor nutrition. The condition may also be linked to untreated HIV/AIDS or other diseases and/or medications that have an immunosuppressive effect, such as chemotherapy or antirejection drugs used in transplant patients.

Periodontitis as a manifestation of systemic disease

The third and final type is where plaque-induced periodontitis is a key feature of a systemic disease (Jepsen et al, 2018). Most of these involve systemic syndromes that impact the immune system, making the patient more susceptible to periodontitis. The management of this kind of periodontitis is still driven by a dysbiotic biofilm, so the focus is on biofilm control. An example of systemic periodontitis is Papillon–Lefèvre syndrome, where the immune system is dysfunctional and the biofilm is not kept in check. Most importantly for us, the dysfunctional immune system rapidly destroys the periodontium.

5.4 Other conditions affecting the periodontium

There are five subcategories under the 'other conditions of the periodontium' section of the classification.

Systemic diseases and conditions affecting the periodontal supporting tissues

These are systemic diseases or conditions that have periodontal manifestations; mostly, these are in the gingivae (eg for Crohn's, sarcoidosis, or herpes simplex) but some affect the periodontal tissues (eg ameloblastoma or chondrosarcoma's histiocytosis) (Jepsen et al, 2018).

Broadly, these disorders can be subdivided into:

- Systemic disorders that have a major impact on the loss of periodontal tissues by influencing periodontal inflammation. These tend to be genetic disorders, acquired immunodeficiency diseases, and inflammatory diseases.

- Other systemic disorders that influence the pathogenesis of periodontal diseases.

- Systemic disorders that can result in loss of periodontal tissues independent of periodontitis – for example, neoplasms, and other disorders that may affect the periodontal tissues.

Periodontal abscesses and endo-perio lesions

A periodontal abscess is a localised collection of pus within the gingival wall of the periodontal pocket or sulcus. It can lead to rapid tissue destruction, jeopardise the prognosis of the affected tooth, and carries a risk of spreading infection systemically. Periodontal abscesses can be subclassified based on their underlying causes.

An endo–perio lesion is a pathological communication between the pulpal and periodontal tissues, which can be either acute or chronic. The main signs are a deep periodontal pocket reaching the root apex and a negative or altered response to pulp sensibility tests. These lesions can be further categorised based on their signs and symptoms, which directly affect their prognosis and treatment (Papapanou et al, 2018).

Mucogingival deformities and conditions

Gingival recession falls under this category, and can be classified as below, as described by Jepsen et al (2018). This will be discussed in more detail later in the book.

- **'Recession Type 1 (RT1):** Gingival recession with no loss of interproximal attachment. Interproximal cementoenamel junction (CEJ) is clinically not detectable at both mesial and distal aspects of the tooth.

- **Recession Type 2 (RT2):** Gingival recession associated with loss of interproximal attachment. The amount of interproximal attachment loss (measured from the interproximal CEJ to the depth of the interproximal sulcus/pocket) is less than or equal to the buccal attachment loss (measured from the buccal CEJ to the apical end of the buccal sulcus/pocket).

- **Recession Type 3 (RT3):** Gingival recession associated with loss of interproximal attachment. The amount of interproximal attachment loss is higher than the buccal attachment loss.'

Traumatic occlusal forces

Traumatic occlusal forces can cause damage to the teeth and the surrounding periodontal structures. Signs of trauma may include increased tooth mobility, adaptive tooth movement (fremitus), an enlarged periodontal ligament space seen on radiographs, tooth migration, pain or discomfort while chewing, and root resorption.

Primary occlusal trauma refers to injury resulting from traumatic occlusal forces exerted on teeth with normal periodontal support, leading to adaptive mobility. By contrast, secondary occlusal trauma occurs when normal or traumatic occlusal forces affect teeth with compromised support, resulting in progressive mobility (Jepsen et al, 2018).

Tooth- and prosthesis-related factors

This subcategory covers tooth anatomical factors, root proximity, abnormalities and fractures, and tooth relationships in the dental arch that are related to dental plaque biofilm-induced gingival inflammation and loss of periodontal supporting tissues (Jepsen et al, 2018).

Dental materials may be associated with hypersensitivity reactions. Clinically these may appear as areas of localised inflammation, unaffected by adequate measures of plaque control. Additional diagnostic measures are usually needed to confirm hypersensitivity.

5.5 Peri-implant diseases and conditions

There are various conditions and diseases that can affect peri-implant tissue; before discussing these though, it's important to understand what optimal peri-implant health looks like.

Peri-implant health

In a state of health, there are no visual differences between the gingivae surrounding natural teeth and implants. However, the probing depths are typically deeper around implant sites versus those of natural teeth (Berglundh et al, 2018). Additionally, the interproximal papillae around implants may be shorter than those found between adjacent teeth.

Clinical methods to detect the presence of inflammation include visual inspection, probing, and digital palpation. It is essential to probe the tissues around implants to evaluate bleeding on probing, and to track any changes in probing depth and mucosal margin migration. There is evidence that probing of the peri-implant tissue using a light probing force is safe and important (Berglundh et al, 2018). While a specific range of probing depths indicative of health cannot be established, the clinical indicators of inflammation carry greater significance. Implants can maintain healthy peri-implant tissues even when there is diminished bone support.

Peri-implant mucositis

Peri-implant mucositis is usually reversible. The key clinical feature of peri-implant mucositis is bleeding on gentle probing, but additional signs may include erythema, swelling, and/or suppuration. Clinical signs of inflammation are required for a diagnosis of peri-implant mucositis. An increase in probing depth is commonly seen in peri-implant mucositis, due to swelling or a reduced resistance during probing. There is strong evidence from both animal and human studies to support the notion that dental plaque is the primary cause of peri-implant mucositis (Berglundh et al, 2018).

Peri-implantitis

Peri-implantitis is an infectious condition that leads to inflammation in the peri-implant mucosa and impacts the surrounding bone (Berglundh et al, 2018). This disease often presents without symptoms, which can leave patients unaware of its progression. If regular maintenance and monitoring visits are not conducted, individuals may experience substantial bone loss before seeking dental care.

Summary of peri-implant conditions

Peri-implant health	• Absence of clinical signs of inflammation
	• Absence of bleeding/ suppuration on gentle probing
	• No increase in probing depth compared to previous examinations
	• No bone loss
Peri-implant mucositis	• Bleeding and/or suppuration on gentle probing
	• No bone loss

Peri-implantitis	• Bleeding and/or suppuration on gentle probing
	• Increased probing depth compared to previous examinations
	• Bone loss

In the absence of previous examination data, a diagnosis of peri-implantitis can be based on the combination of:

     • Bleeding and/or suppuration on gentle probing

     • Probing depths of ≥ 6 mm

     • Bone levels ≥ 3 mm apical of the most coronal portion of the intra-osseous part of the implant

6
Prognosis

Prognostic setting should be the next step following your diagnosis (or diagnoses). It is also a prerequisite for drawing up your treatment plan.

6.1 Importance and details

Establishing a prognosis involves predicting the trajectory and outcome of a particular disease, as well as the likelihood of recovery. When a prognosis is provided, the aim is to anticipate how a tooth or multiple teeth will react to treatment over time, taking into account all factors that could influence the results.

From a medico-legal perspective, it is crucial for patients to be informed about prognoses. Often, claims arise from patients saying they were not told that a particular tooth was at risk of being lost in the future. From a clinical point of view, this prognostic awareness can facilitate better decision-making during the treatment planning process for both short- and long-term care.

Determining the prognosis of individual teeth can be difficult due to the multiple factors that influence treatment outcomes, but a thorough history, identification of risk factors, detailed examination, and appropriate radiographs will be important here.

The factors that need to be considered when determining a tooth's prognosis can be divided into patient factors and local factors (Mordohai et al, 2007).

The patient factors include:

1. Risk factors – such as diabetes, smoking, stress, and nutrition

2. Compliance with oral hygiene and maintenance

While the local factors are:

1. Probing depth and the tooth position – for example, the prognosis of an incisor with probing depths of 5 mm will be far better than the prognosis of a molar with a 10 mm pocket.

2. Furcation involvement – less favourable outcomes have been shown for furcation-involved teeth, especially when Grade 2 or 3. Maxillary molars with furcation involvement usually have poorer prognoses than mandibular molars with furcation involvement.

3. Amount of bone loss – advanced bone loss has been reported to be associated with greater future bone loss and reduced survival rates when bone loss is over 75%. The amount of bone loss will also affect the crown-to-root ratio and, if it is unsatisfactory, this may affect the prognosis.

4. Anatomical defects, such as cervical enamel projections, enamel pearls, and root grooves, are all local factors that may negatively affect the prognosis.

5. Other associated pathology.

6.2 Prognostic systems

Several attempts have been made to devise prognostic classification schemes and criteria. Although there is no accepted system for determining a prognosis, and it is recognised that a high level of subjective clinical judgement is involved, some common terms or categories can be used (Nibali et al, 2016).

A commonly used prognostic system is good, fair, guarded, and hopeless. Sometimes, 'questionable' or 'poor' are used instead of 'guarded'. A more simplified approach could be to use favourable, uncertain, and unfavourable. This can be broken down as follows:

- **Favourable** is when there is no evidence of disease or mild disease, and you are likely to get an optimal result from treatment. There are no major risk factors or local factors. The patient's oral hygiene is optimal, and they appear to have a good level of compliance.

- **Uncertain** is when you are unsure how the tooth will respond to treatment. The level of disease is moderate, and there may be risk factors or local factors involved.

- **Unfavourable** teeth are not likely to respond to treatment and will need to be extracted now or in the future. If asymptomatic and not causing damage to neighbouring teeth, patients may wish to hold onto unfavourable teeth until they cause issues.

A tooth-by-tooth prognosis is common practice when seeing a periodontal patient, especially those with more severe disease. But on occasion, for speed, you might want to group teeth together; for example, you might observe that, 'all of the molars have uncertain prognoses.' Strictly speaking, there is also a difference between the periodontal prognosis and the overall prognosis so, if needed, you can split these up.

Prognostic setting is completed at the initial stage, prior to treatment. However, it may be adjusted after initial treatment once a full appreciation of the individual's healing potential, compliance, and susceptibility can be gained. Risk factors might also change during initial treatment. Therefore, you might want to add a statement after your prognoses explaining that they 'may change at the reassessment stage.'

PART THREE
THE MANAGEMENT

7
Treatment Planning

The European Federation of Periodontology has issued the latest (EFP S3) guidelines on treatment planning and management. They are evidence and consensus-based and cover the management of Stage I–III (Sanz et al, 2020) and Stage IV periodontitis (Herrera et al, 2022). The British Society of Periodontology has released an implementation paper to guide the application of these guidelines to UK practice (West et al, 2021).

In these guidelines, a sequence of treatments is discussed, commencing with the basis of therapy – examination, assessment of risk factors, and diagnosis. The advice is to inform the patient of their diagnosis, including the causes of their condition, risk factors, treatment alternatives, and expected risks and benefits, including the option of no treatment. This is a crucial conversation that can easily be glossed over in a busy general practice setting.

This should be followed by an agreement on a personalised care plan. The emphasis here is that every patient requires a bespoke plan that suits their needs. This plan may require adjustments throughout the treatment process based on the patient's preferences, clinical observations, and any changes in their overall health.

7.1 The stepwise approach

Commonly, dental professionals will apply the stepwise approach to treatment planning, which consists of four steps:

1. Supragingival PMPR and risk factor control

2. Subgingival PMPR

3. Repeat subgingival PMPR or surgery

4. Supportive periodontal care

Step 1

Step 1 focuses on establishing a solid foundation for effective treatment and ongoing maintenance. This involves providing thorough oral hygiene instructions and facilitating behavioural changes. Efforts are made to manage modifiable risk factors as effectively as possible, and supragingival PMPR is performed.

PMPR = professional mechanical plaque removal

The term PMPR refers to professional mechanical plaque removal, and this replaces all other historic terminology (Sanz et al, 2020). PMPR can be divided into supragingival PMPR (carried out in Steps 1 and 4) or subgingival PMPR (Steps 2, 3, 4).

The key expert consensus-based recommendations from the guidelines include (West et al, 2021):

- The same oral hygiene guidance to control gingival inflammation should be practised throughout Steps 1–4 of periodontal therapy.

- Supragingival PMPR and control of biofilm / plaque-retentive factors as part of the first step of therapy.

- As part of the first step of therapy in periodontitis patients, risk factor control interventions (eg for diabetes and smoking) should be completed.

Step 2

The second step focuses on cause-related therapy once the patient is engaged. 'Engagement' has been defined as:

- $\geq 50\%$ improvement in plaque and marginal bleeding scores, or

- Plaque levels $\leq 20\%$ and bleeding levels $\leq 30\%$, or

- The patient has met targets outlined in their personal self-care plan, as determined by their dentist

A detailed periodontal pocket and bleeding chart should be completed prior to subgingival PMPR.

The key expert consensus-based recommendations for Step 2, taken from the guidelines, include (West et al, 2021):

- Subgingival PMPR should be employed to treat periodontitis in order to reduce gingival inflammation, the number of diseased sites, and probing pocket depths.

- Subgingival PMPR should be performed with hand or powered (sonic/ultrasonic) instruments, either alone or in combination.

- Subgingival PMPR can be performed using a traditional quadrant-wise approach or full-mouth delivery using a one- or two-stage technique within a twenty-four-hour period.

- It is suggested that lasers are not used as adjuncts to subgingival instrumentation.

- It is suggested that adjunctive antimicrobial photodynamic therapy is not used in patients with periodontitis.

- Adjuncts to mechanical debridement may be considered in specific cases, including antiseptics for a limited period, or systemic antibiotics. Systemic antibiotics may be considered for specific patient categories, for example, Grade C.

Step 3

After completing Step 2, the patient's treatment response is assessed. If the patient is still unstable, meaning the endpoints of therapy have not been met, additional treatment will be initiated. Conversely, if the patient is stable and the treatment goals have been successfully achieved, they will transition to a supportive periodontal care programme.

For patients who are engaged, further treatment options may be available, including both non-surgical and surgical procedures (such as access flap, resective, or regenerative techniques). Typically, surgery is not recommended following just one phase of non-surgical treatment. At this point, a referral to a complexity level 2 or 3 clinician may be necessary. If a referral isn't feasible, options include repeating subgingival PMPR or placing the patient on supportive periodontal care (likely palliative). Further discussion regarding surgical options will be provided in Part Four of this book.

Step 4

Supportive periodontal care (SPC) is essential for preserving periodontal stability and is recommended for all patients who have undergone treatment for periodontitis. Patients should be informed about SPC prior to commencing their treatment plan, otherwise they are likely to assume that once active treatment is complete, they are 'cured'. This can lead to unhappy patients and potential medico-legal complaints. SPC may incorporate both preventive and therapeutic measures from Steps 1 and 2. The frequency of SPC appointments will be customised to meet the individual needs of each patient. If signs of recurrent disease are identified, re-treatment will be necessary, and a new diagnosis and treatment plan should be established.

The key expert consensus-based recommendations from the guidelines include (West et al, 2021):

- SPC visits should be scheduled for intervals of three months to a maximum of twelve months, with the frequency determined by the patient's risk profile and periodontal status after active therapy.

- When selecting a toothbrush and design of interdental brush, the patient's abilities, needs, preferences, and manual dexterity must be considered.

- For patients receiving SPC, tooth brushing should be supplemented by the use of interdental brushes (where anatomically possible).

- Flossing is not the first-choice method of interdental cleaning for SPC patients.

- The use of other interdental cleaning devices in interdental areas, not reachable by interdental brushes, may be considered when receiving SPC.

- If an antiseptic mouth rinse formulation is to be considered for the adjunctive control of gingival inflammation for patients under SPC, use of products that contain chlorhexidine, essential oils, or cetylpyridinium chloride are suggested.

7.2 A typical treatment plan

Below is a template for a typical treatment plan for a patient with periodontitis:

1. Discussion of the importance of optimal diabetes control (if relevant).

2. Smoking or vaping cessation (if relevant).

3. Oral hygiene instructions – brushing technique using an electric toothbrush, use of a single-tufted brush, and daily use of appropriately sized interdental brushes.

4. Full six-point pocket chart.

5. Full-mouth supragingival PMPR.

6. Subgingival PMPR for probing depths of 4 mm or more with bleeding, or more than 5 mm under local anaesthesia – quadrant by quadrant/half-mouth/full-mouth approach.

7. Reassessment eight weeks later, and further treatment planning.

8. Lifelong supportive periodontal care on a three-monthly basis.

7.3 Working as a team

When treating patients with periodontitis in practice, it can be helpful to devise a practice protocol and decide which team member will focus on which treatment step. Everyone should be singing from the same hymn book – for example, BPEs should not be drastically different between team members. Inconsistencies can lead to patient confusion and medico-legal issues.

Hygienists/therapists form an integral part of the team, and dentists should be aware of any requirements when working with them. If the hygienist/therapist will be completing the treatment and providing the majority of the care, it's preferred that the hygienist/therapist decide on the number of visits required and set the recall interval as needed.

7.4 Referral

The British Society of Periodontology has provided guidelines on patient referrals (BSP, 2020). Referral of patients with periodontal diseases to specialists or other appropriately qualified dental professionals depends on several factors:

- The stage and grade of disease, as well as the complexity of treatment required

- The patient's desire to see a specialist or undergo specialist treatment

- The knowledge, experience, and training of oral healthcare professionals to manage patients with a range of periodontal conditions

- The presence of genetic and lifestyle/behavioural risk factors

The BSP (2020) has outlined guidance for complexity levels 2 and 3.

Level 2 complexity

Treatment for conditions at this level can typically be managed by oral healthcare professionals within a general dental practice, although referrals may sometimes be necessary. In certain cases, periodontal or peri-implant treatments might need to be provided by a specialist as part of a more intricate, integrated treatment plan. This category includes patients with Stage II, III, or IV periodontitis who have residual true pocketing of 6 mm or more following initial periodontal therapy; Grade C periodontitis determined by a specialist; or complexities such as furcation defects and challenging root morphologies, especially when these are strategically important and delegated by a specialist.

For conditions such as gingival enlargement, non-surgical management in collaboration with medical professionals may be necessary. Pocket reduction surgery may be included in this category, especially when delegated by a specialist. Furthermore, certain non-plaque-induced periodontal diseases, such as those induced by viral infections, autoimmune disorders, abnormal pigmentation, vesiculobullous disease, or periodontal manifestations of gastrointestinal and other systemic conditions, should be managed here under specialist guidance. Peri-implant mucositis also falls within this complexity level.

Level 3 complexity

Patients at this level are usually referred after lifestyle or behavioural risk factors have been addressed and appropriate non-surgical treatments have been completed in a general practice setting. Conditions at this level include Grade C or Stage IV periodontitis and true pocketing of 6 mm or more. Cases requiring periodontal surgery will fall under this category. Furcation defects and other complex root morphologies that are unsuitable for delegation must also be managed by a specialist. Additionally, non-plaque-induced periodontal diseases that are not suitable for management by a practitioner with enhanced skills require specialist care.

Patients who need multidisciplinary care should be referred to a specialist. Furthermore, if patients with level 2 complexity do not respond to treatment, they may need to be re-evaluated and referred to this complexity. For non-plaque-induced periodontal diseases, a differential diagnosis should be established, and joint care pathways should be developed in collaboration with relevant medical colleagues. In some cases, it may be necessary to manage these conditions collaboratively with practitioners with enhanced skills. Specialists may also provide advice and assist with treatment planning for colleagues. Finally, cases involving peri-implantitis require specialist attention.

Patients with modifying factors, particularly those for whom behaviour change is difficult, may need to be escalated to a higher level of care. Those diagnosed with Grade C periodontitis should be referred for further treatment following initial preventive guidance on managing risk factors and oral hygiene instruction.

The modifying factors that are outlined in the BSP (2020) guidance include:

- 'Coordinated medical or dental multi-disciplinary care

- Regular tobacco smoking and tobacco substitute products that deliver nicotine, eg vaping

- Dental special care for the acceptance or provision of treatment

- Concurrent mucogingival disease, eg erosive lichen planus

- Medical history that significantly affects clinical management, eg:

  - Patients with a history of head / neck radiotherapy or intravenous bisphosphonate therapy

  - Patients who are significantly immunocompromised or immunosuppressed

  - Patients with a significant bleeding dyscrasia / disorder

  - Patients with a potential drug interaction'

Not referring at an appropriate time is a common reason for litigation. It's also much easier for patients to allege, after the event (usually loss of a tooth), that they would have preferred a referral for specialist care. Therefore, it's important to minimise any delay in referral.

8
Educating And
Empowering Patients

Achieving success in periodontal treatment is a team sport and the patient is at the centre of this. Educating patients is imperative to ensure they understand their condition and what the treatment will involve. Patients also need to take on responsibility for their condition and understand that much of the success in treatment will be down to what they do at home.

In this chapter, we will discuss how to communicate clinical findings to the patient as well as the benefits of treatment. We will then explore the key steps for effective home care and behaviour change.

8.1 Translating the clinical findings and treatment plan

There are various clinical findings that will need to be communicated and explained in a way that both makes sense to the patient and motivates them to take responsibility for maintaining oral health at home. The main things you will need to discuss with patients are pockets and bleeding, your diagnoses, and the proposed treatment plan. It's essential that patients understand all these elements in order to maximise chances of successful treatment.

Pockets and bleeding

A pocket can be explained as the space between the tooth and gum that opens and deepens as the disease of periodontitis progresses. It's helpful to use the phrase 'open pocket' for any site that requires active treatment, ie that has probing depths of 4 mm with bleeding or 5 mm and above. A 'closed pocket' does not require active treatment, ie probing depths of 4 mm and below without bleeding. If the patient wants more detail, you can mention that probing depths of 1–3 mm is considered healthy, 4–5 mm is moderate, and 6 mm and above indicates severe disease. Highlighting all the 'open pockets' on your pocket chart can be a useful way to help the patient visualise the disease extent. This can then be used as a comparison following treatment.

When discussing bleeding, it is key to emphasise that bleeding is not normal and is an alarm bell in the body. For example, you could say, 'We wouldn't ignore bleeding from any other part of our body, so we shouldn't ignore bleeding from our gums.' It is useful to separate gingival/marginal bleeding (related to suboptimal home care) from bleeding on probing (a sign of active disease). When you are explaining your findings from the pocket chart, you can use simplistic terms like 'outside bleeding' if they mention their gums are bleeding on brushing, ie gingival bleeding, and 'inside bleeding', ie bleeding on probing.

Radiographic findings

Always explain to the patients that radiographs are required to check the bone levels around their teeth. If they are reluctant for you to take radiographs, ask them, 'Would you let a mechanic fix your car without lifting the hood? The same applies here; we need to see under the gum to be able to diagnose and fix the issue.'

Radiographs are an excellent way to evidence to patients the damage that has occurred through periodontitis. Show the patient where their bone level should be, where it is now, and the end of the root. Radiographs are also helpful for showing calculus and other local factors, such as overhangs. If appropriate, root anatomy can form a part of the conversation in terms of anchorage. For example, for someone with short conical roots, the impact of 50% bone loss may be more significant than if the roots were long and tapered.

Diagnosis

Medico-legally, patients need to know their periodontal diagnosis. Gum disease is easy to understand, but it is still useful to use the technically correct phrase, so gingivitis or periodontitis. The severity also needs to be discussed; you may want to mention mild/moderate/severe or the stage of their condition. Their grading can be considered as a marker of the patient's susceptibility as well as the rate of future disease progression without treatment. For example, with a patient who is Grade C, you can emphasise that they are highly susceptible and that, without treatment, there is a high risk of tooth loss.

As well as the diagnosis, it's worth talking about why the patient has the condition, ie the risk factors, and the consequences of not treating it, such as tooth loss and a potential impact on general health.

Treatment plan

To ensure the best chances of treatment uptake and compliance, it's important to translate the treatment plan and focus on what matters to the patient. For instance, explaining that the treatment will 'improve probing depths' may not be relatable; these clinical outcomes are important to us but not necessarily to the patient. On the other hand, mentioning that, with treatment, they will keep their teeth for longer, may not have to wear dentures, or wake up with blood on their pillow may be more impactful. Focus on patient-related factors that impact quality of life – the patient may have mentioned what is bothering them during their initial presenting complaint, so link back to that. Even when the patient's condition is severe, keep as positive a spin as possible when communicating the plan and focus on the good news: you can do something to help them (even if a few teeth may need to be sacrificed in the process).

8.2 Essential steps for effective home care

As periodontitis is a multifactorial inflammatory disease associated with dysbiotic dental plaque biofilms, optimal biofilm control through effective home care is the cornerstone of the prevention and treatment of periodontal diseases. It is the first and most powerful step of therapy, aimed at guiding behaviour change by empowering and motivating the patient to successfully remove or disrupt supragingival biofilm.

Time is often limited in practice, so it's helpful to follow a structure or framework to maximise efficiency and effectiveness when providing oral hygiene instructions for patients to apply at home. I recommend a five-step process: orientate, disclose, demonstrate, reinforce responsibility, and apply the GPS model.

Step 1: Orientate

- Patients are generally unfamiliar with their oral anatomy and have an inadequate spatial sense, so begin by introducing the basic anatomy of the oral tissues. The teeth and gingivae can be visualised using a mirror or intraoral camera.

- Pull the patient's lower lip down and show them, using a probe, where the tooth is, where the gumline is, and where the pocket is. Explain that the pocket is where 'bugs' get trapped, and that's why the toothbrush needs to be angled in that direction, towards the gums.

- Radiographs can be helpful in showing areas of calculus and spaces that need to be cleaned.

Step 2: Disclose

- Use a disclosing tablet/sponge/liquid to highlight to the patient areas they are missing during their brushing. This will allow you to provide more tailored advice.

- Disclosing allows you to gain an accurate, objective plaque score as a percentage rather than a subjective statement such as 'oral hygiene is good/fair/poor.'

- Inform the patient of their score, as this can be a great motivational tool for improving compliance. Patients should be aiming for low percentages of plaque. However, if the patient is a child, it may be helpful to flip this to percentage plaque-free to make it more motivational, as children strive to score high numbers.

- Taking a photo for the patient on their camera phone is a great idea, as they can refer to it easily between visits.

Step 3: Demonstrate

- Set up a reminder system to request that the patient bring their oral hygiene aids to their appointments. Ask them first to demonstrate what they are doing and then adapt as needed.

- Allowing the patient to demonstrate what they're doing at home will allow you to pick up if they have any manual dexterity issues due to medical conditions, including arthritis. If this is the case, always advise an electric toothbrush with a decent-sized handle. If using a manual toothbrush, you can suggest they use putty around the handle to help with the grip.

- Demonstrating correct technique in their mouth will be more helpful than using models, as the feel component is important. Test drive electric toothbrushes from the key manufacturers should be used.

- Ask the patient to video you showing them brushing and interdental cleaning techniques in their mouth, as this can be a helpful reminder for those needing extra guidance. Tailored oral hygiene leaflets can also help reinforce all instructions.

- For those patients constantly missing areas, ask them to start there first, as patients are more likely to have the most energy and do a better job at the start of their oral hygiene regime.

- Keep it simple and repeat/reinforce the advice at each visit.

Step 4: Reinforce the patient's responsibility

- Emphasise to the patient that the outcome of the treatment plan is 80% about what they do at home and 20% about what we do. A shift in mindset where they take ownership of their condition is key for both short- and long-term success.

Step 5: GPS

GPS is an evidence-based technique that can help achieve behavioural change (Tonetti et al, 2015), where G stands for goal setting, P is for planning, and S is for self-monitoring. Below is an example of how you can apply it in your practice:

- **Goal:** 'Today we found your plaque score was 80%, let's try and reduce this to 40%.'

- **Planning:** 'We can do this by just focusing on the brushing technique we went through today. We can then review how you're doing in two to three weeks.'

- **Self-monitoring:** 'I'm going to give you some of these plaque-disclosing tablets. I want you to use them every week. Carry out your usual home care regime, then use the tablet. Wherever you see the pink/purple staining, go back and clean those areas. You should notice them decrease with time, which means you're getting better.'

The last step in particular is extremely powerful and crucial to treatment success.

8.3 Behavioural change

To understand our role in guiding behavioural change and motivating patients, it's useful to compare the dental professional's role to that of a personal trainer. We are there to guide them, but the patient must ultimately put in the work. A daily timetable with time carved out for oral care is key. For our part, we need to appreciate that behavioural change is not easy but should reassure the patient that it does get easier with practice, and their enjoyment of it may increase when the benefits become clearer. We must provide honest feedback during the patient's journey while rewarding positive performance.

Several behavioural change models have been proposed for the field of dentistry. Oral Hygiene TIPPS from the Scottish Dental Effectiveness Programme aims to make patients feel more confident in their ability to perform effective biofilm removal and help them plan how and when they will look after their teeth and gums. Key steps include:

- **Talk** with the patient about the causes of periodontal disease and discuss any barriers to effective biofilm removal.

- **Instruct** the patient on the best ways to perform effective biofilm removal.

- Ask the patient to **practise** cleaning his/her teeth and to use the interdental cleaning aids while in the dental surgery.

- Put in place a **plan** that specifies how the patient will incorporate oral hygiene into their daily life.

- Provide **support** to the patient by following up at subsequent visits.

Alternatively the COM-B model of behaviour change model suggests that capability (C), opportunity (O), and motivation (M) are essential for any behaviour (B) to change (Michie et al, 2011).

When the patient lacks motivation, it's important to focus on patient-derived change to ensure realistic steps forward. The aim here is to connect change with what the patient values and ask them to come up with practical goals.

8.4 Key recommendations

Any specific recommendations you make should consider the patient's abilities, preferences, and needs (Sanz et al, 2020).

Brushes

Advise power brushes (specifically rechargeable oscillating-rotating) over manual toothbrushes where possible, as these have been shown to be more effective in reducing plaque levels (Yaacob et al, 2014). Focused gum brushing is key, angling the brush 45 degrees to the axes of the teeth, with the end of the filaments pointing into the gingival crevice. The timer and pressure indicator on the rechargeable brushes are helpful prompts for the patient. For the rechargeable brush, it's important to ensure the patient is not using this like a manual brush but rather holding it against the tooth/gum for three seconds or so before moving on to the next tooth. Tell the patient the brush 'is doing the work for you.' Brushing twice a day is important.

Interdental brushes are the first choice for interdental cleaning (Slot et al, 2020). The correct size is key, so it can be helpful to check these for patients and emphasise the need for a snug fit. During the active treatment phase, these sizes may change. Interdental cleaning should be carried out at least once a day before toothbrushing, and interdental brushes usually need replacing every few days.

If the interdental brushes don't fit, floss is recommended. To be effective, the floss needs to be correctly adapted to the tooth surface by gently wrapping it around the tooth once past the contact site. Use of floss holders can make flossing easier.

Single-tufted brushes are popular amongst patients with periodontitis to help address hard to reach areas. This may include distal and lingually around molars, crowded areas, localised recession defects and in those with a sensitive gag reflex. The single-tufted brush is best used with a pen grip using the push, splay, wiggle technique.

Other tools

Oral irrigators or water flossers may be helpful for those patients who are struggling with the above, but the evidence for their clinical efficacy is sparse comparatively. Some patients may be keen to use these in addition to other interdental cleaning.

Tongue cleaning is recommended, especially if there is a tongue coating. This would be the final step in someone's oral hygiene regime, likely once a day.

When a patient asks you to recommend specific products, it's worth having your key one in mind, depending on their symptoms, to prevent extensive discussion and loss of time during appointments. Your chosen product may be related to the current evidence base and your patient's experience. Having a product prescription table (like the below) to hand that you can update regularly may be helpful.

Example product prescription table

Symptom	Prescription
Bad breath	*Insert chosen product here*
Sensitivity	*Insert chosen product here*
Sore gums	*Insert chosen product here*
No problems	*Insert chosen product here*

Sustainability

Patients may mention that they don't want to use certain brushes due to the plastic wastage. It's important to emphasise that they can still be eco-friendly without compromising their health. Plastic-free options do exist for interdental brushes, but these may not always be of the appropriate size. Instead, encourage recycling. There are specific oral hygiene recycling boxes, and these can be housed in the dental practice so that patients can bring any items they'd like to recycle with them each time they visit.

8.5 Oral hygiene analogies

Analogies can be helpful ways to communicate the importance of oral hygiene to patients that avoid off-putting technical or medical terminology that they might not engage with. Below are some examples you could consider using:

- Toothpaste is like face cream. You pick your cream depending on your skin type. It's the same for teeth. For example, if you have sensitive teeth, you might need a toothpaste that is targeted to address sensitivity, or if you have no issues, you just need a regular fluoride toothpaste.

- Regular mouthwash is like perfume after a shower. You don't usually need it and there are no added health benefits unless it's been specifically recommended by your dental professional.

- If you don't clean in between your teeth, it's like only cleaning one side of your plate and then eating from it again. All surfaces need to be thoroughly cleaned.

- If you had a life-threatening condition and you were told to take an important medication daily, you would. Look at interdental brushes the same way; they are super important and should just become part of your routine.

- Oral irrigators or water flossers are not replacements for interdental brushes. They are adjuncts, if you want to use them. If you had a dirty dish that needed washing, using these devices is like just rinsing the dish, but what you would really need to do to get the dish properly clean is scrub. That's what the interdental brushes do.

- The tongue is like a carpet – if it's not vacuumed, debris will build up and it will smell. In the same way, the tongue needs to be cleaned regularly.

8.6 Biofilm-retentive factors

Biofilm-retentive factors can be considered as local risk factors for disease initiation and progression, as they increase the likelihood that oral hygiene will be compromised and that biofilm will accumulate. These should be assessed and addressed where possible. Examples include anatomical and caries and iatrogenic factors.

Anatomical factors

- Tooth position (crowding, teeth out of alignment, teeth out of function, loss of contact points)

- Gingival anatomy (recession, high frenal attachments)

- Tooth anatomy (bulbosity of teeth, marginal ridges, abnormalities such as enamel pearls, and *dens in dente*)

- Root anatomy (furcations, root fissures/fossas/ grooves)

Caries and iatrogenic factors

- Carious cavities

- Poorly designed restorations (lack of contact points, poor margins, rough finish, lack of marginal ridge, poor contour, poor design)

- Removable prostheses and appliances

9
Non-Surgical Periodontal Therapy

As discussed in Chapter 7, the patient must be engaged before commencing non-surgical periodontal therapy. Active treatment is required in probing depths of 4 mm with bleeding on probing or 5 mm and above. The aim is to 'close' the pocket – to achieve probing depths of 4 mm (without bleeding on probing) or below. Pocket depth reduction will occur by a combination of gingival recession, long-junctional epithelium formation, as well as resolution of gingival inflammation and cuff tightening. The true endpoints of non-surgical periodontal therapy are an improvement in tooth prognosis, a reduction in systemic inflammation and a positive impact on the patient's quality of life.

It's important to be aware of expected improvements so that if these are not achieved, you can investigate the factors at play before considering further active treatment.

These are the improvements we would expect to see from non-surgical therapy (Suvan, 2020):

- For shallow sites (probing depths of 5 mm or less) the mean reduction is 1.5 mm after three months and 1.6 mm after six to eight months.

- For deep sites (probing depths of 7 mm or more) the mean reduction is 2.6 mm after three months and 2.6 mm after six to eight months.

Tomasi et al (2022) highlight that pocket closure is most predictable around anterior teeth and least likely around molar teeth. Furthermore, the higher the initial probing depth, the lower the likelihood of pocket closure.

Do not underestimate the power of good-quality non-surgical periodontal therapy; according to Suvan (2020), 74% of pockets can be treated non-surgically.

9.1 Consent

Written consent for non-surgical periodontal therapy is not essential but verbal consent following a discussion is. The patient must be aware of the treatment proposed, what is involved, and the benefits. When exploring side effects and risks, the four key areas to discuss include:

1. **Pain:** Explain that some soreness is not uncommon, but it can usually be managed with the same analgesia they would take for a headache.

2. **Bleeding:** Bleeding on toothbrushing or use of interdental brushes may initially increase before it settles down. Ensure this doesn't put the patient off their self-care regime.

3. **Sensitivity:** While frequently occurring, sensitivity is most often short-term. Advise the use of a toothpaste for sensitivity, ensuring the patient spits and doesn't rinse it out.

4. **Gum recession:** As healing occurs and swelling reduces, gingival recession may occur. The patient needs to be aware that this is a good sign, and long-term management options can be discussed following stability if it bothers them.

9.2 Local anaesthesia

When completing subgingival PMPR, local anaesthesia can be helpful to ensure maximum patient comfort and the most effective instrumentation. Being able to provide local anaesthesia comfortably is an important skill to develop. Here are a few tips and tricks to help:

- Create a calming environment by avoiding phrases like, 'This will hurt a bit,' or 'This will feel uncomfortable,' and try to use positive language like 'You're doing great, we are more than halfway through' instead. Ensure the needle/syringe isn't within view of the patient.

- Manage the patient's psychological state by providing them with a control signal, asking them to focus on their breathing, and using tools like music as a distraction.

- One of the most discomfort-inducing steps in delivering local anaesthesia is the penetration of the needle through the most superficial tissues. To reduce this, you can use topical anaesthesia in the form of a concentrated solution, gel, or spray that is applied to the mucosa. Ensure this is left on for at least one minute before inserting the needle.

- Pressure adjacent to the injection site using a firm but dull object (eg a mirror or cotton bud) can be a helpful distraction. Gently shaking the mirror in the sulcus can also be a useful way of distracting the patient.

- Blunt needles can cause pain, so only use sharp needles. If you are completing more than one quadrant, perhaps have two needles ready on the tray. Always direct the needle bevel towards the bone.

- Ensure the anaesthetic solution is at room temperature or above. To prevent discomfort, it is wise to allow refrigerated cartridges to warm to room temperature prior to use.

- Once the needle has penetrated the mucosa, the main sensation of discomfort felt by the patient is due to the deposition of the solution. Deposition over a longer period helps to prevent discomfort, and patients tend to show fewer signs of pain.

- If not using traditional blocks, try and inject where already numb – once you've provided the first infiltration, the area around that point will be anaesthetised. Try and make your next injection point in that same area and the patient is unlikely to feel it. Then keep working back or forward. A popular choice of anaesthetic for periodontal procedures is 4% articaine + 1:100,000 adrenaline, which can be used as infiltrations across the mouth.

- Make the most of technology such as The Wand, which is a computer-controlled local anaesthesia delivery device.

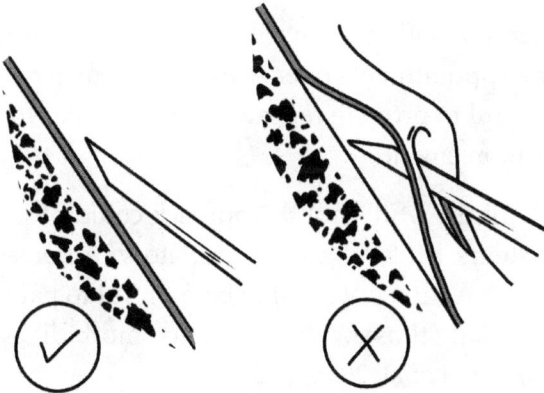

When providing local anaesthesia, the bevel of the needle should be facing the bone to reduce discomfort

9.3 Full/half/quadrant approach

According to the latest treatment guidelines (Sanz et al, 2020), in terms of clinical treatment outcomes, there would appear to be no significant difference between quadrant or full-mouth approaches. How the treatment/appointments are divided will usually depend on other factors, including:

- The severity and extent of the disease.

- Time available per appointment as well as the available patient time.

- Use of local anaesthesia.

- Anxiety – to be discussed with patient, as some anxious patients prefer shorter, more frequent appointments and others prefer one longer appointment.

- Plaque/biofilm score – if not optimal, splitting the appointments over several visits may be helpful to provide repeated opportunities for reinforcement.

- Medical – a full-mouth approach could produce a systemic acute-phase inflammatory response that may have the potential to be harmful to patients, especially those with vascular co-morbidities (Graziani et al, 2015, 2023).

9.4 Adjuncts

As per the discussion in Chapter 7, according to the S3 clinical guidelines (Sanz et al, 2020), there may be a place for specific adjuncts in conjunction with active treatment.

CHX

Chlorhexidine (CHX) mouth rinse may be used for a limited time in specific cases, such as a patient with significant marginal inflammation that is preventing them from completing an adequate oral hygiene regime at home (Da Costa et al, 2017). The guideline also confirms that locally delivered sustained-release chlorhexidine could be considered in patients with periodontitis, though the clinical benefits remain small, equivalent to a pocket reduction effect of approximately 10% (Sanz et al, 2020).

KEY FACTS ABOUT CHX

- It is a biguanide.
- The most common formulation is as a mouthwash (0.2% or 0.12% w/v).
- It's been shown to be the most efficacious mouthwash in clinical trials – antibacterial, antiviral and antifungal. It has an anti-plaque effect which produces a prolonged and profound reduction in plaque sufficient to prevent the development of gingivitis.

- The effectiveness of this drug relies on its ability to reach the cell walls, a process aided by electrostatic interactions. CHX, which is positively charged, binds to the negatively charged bacterial cell walls, specifically targeting phosphate and carboxyl groups. This binding disrupts the osmotic barrier and hampers membrane transport. CHX also adheres well to tooth surfaces and the oral mucosa.
- Indications: unable to carry out mechanical plaque control, before/following surgery, immunocompromised, recurrent aphthous ulceration.
- Unwanted effects: staining of teeth/restorations/tongue, taste disturbances, mucosal desquamation, parotid enlargement, and allergy.

Antibiotics

Use of systemic antibiotics should be limited, as there is a balance to be found between the benefits and risk of antimicrobial resistance (Herrera et al, 2020). Patients with Grade C periodontitis might benefit (Sanz et al, 2020), but in general practice this will only be for a limited number of patients, as patients with Grade C disease are likely to be referred for specialist care. Other examples include those with necrotising periodontitis. Antibiotics should always be used as an adjunct (not alone) and following the last session of subgingival PMPR. Options for periodontitis may include:

- Azithromycin 500 mg, once a day for three days

- Metronidazole 400 mg and Amoxicillin 500 mg, three times a day for five days

- Doxycyline 200 mg (loading dose), 100 mg once a day for fourteen days

Azithromycin is a popular choice, due to the high chance of patient compliance as only one tablet is required per day over three days.

9.5 MINST

Non-surgical periodontal therapy has evolved over the last few decades, moving towards a less invasive and more personalised approach. Minimally invasive non-surgical therapy (MINST) is a novel approach to non-surgical periodontal therapy focused on biofilm removal without intentional loss of tooth structure alongside minimal soft tissue trauma to allow optimal clot stabilisation for wound healing (Nibali et al, 2019).

MINST is used particularly for intrabony defects to optimise healing by avoiding intentionally making the root surfaces smooth and minimising trauma through use of magnification, slimline ultrasonic tips, and mini curettes. This technique aims to stimulate the formation of a stable blood clot, by natural filling of the intrabony defect with blood following debridement, allowing for potential regeneration. As well as allowing for both clinical and radiographic improvement, even in advanced cases, benefits also include reduced patient morbidity, a decreased chance of needing surgery, and saved expense/time (Mehta et al, 2024; Nibali et al, 2019). If site-specific MINST is completed, then reassessment probing should be delayed until around six months.

9.6 Ultrasonics, hand instrumentation, and other devices

In general, no significant difference has been shown between the use of hand and powered instrumentation in terms of deposit removal and improved clinical parameters (Badersten et al, 1981; Loos et al, 1987; Sanz, 2020), but in furcation Grade II or III lesions, powered instruments are more effective due to the difference in tip size (Drisko, 1998). There are specific benefits of both ultrasonic and hand scaling, and so the use of a blended approach is ideal for non-surgical periodontal therapy (Cobb, 1996). A suggested order of use would be ultrasonic followed by hand followed by ultrasonic.

Ultrasonics

Ultrasonics are a type of powered scaler that can be magnetostrictive or piezoelectric. The two kinds work in different ways. In piezoelectric scalers, electrical energy activates ceramic crystals in the handpiece. In magnetostrictive scalers, electrical energy is applied to stacked metal strips and the magnetic field causes metal stacks to elongate and return to normal length, creating vibrations that travel from body to tip.

Ultrasonics have a few key mechanisms of action:

1. **Mechanical:** Vibratory action of the oscillating metal tip against the deposit that ablates the deposit.

2. **Irrigation:** Lavage action of water flowing over the tip flushes biofilm from the tooth's surface.

3. **Cavitation:** Disruption of biofilm by shock waves resulting from implosion of bubbles.

4. **Acoustic microstreaming:** Disruption of biofilm by turbulent currents of water surrounding the tip.

Some top tips on good ultrasonic technique:

- Maintain a light, feather-like touch to maximise tactile sensation

- Adapt 2–4 mm of the active tip area and maintain a 0–15-degree angulation from the long axis of the tooth

- Utilise short, overlapping strokes in a methodical pattern

- Use the lowest effective power setting and increase as required

- Pick the most appropriate tip for the tooth surface in question

- Inserts should be activated prior to insertion into pockets

- Strokes should initiate at the gingival margin

- Piezoelectric – only use lateral surface

- Magnetostrictive – can use all sides

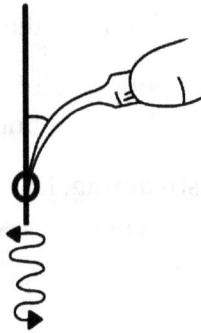

The position of the ultrasonic tip and the use of short overlapping strokes in an erasing motion

One of the most common reasons for ineffective ultrasonic instrumentation is worn-down tips. Wear guides are available from the manufacturers, so regular auditing and replacement of instruments as required is key. If the tip of the handpiece is overheating, check that the water levels have been properly adjusted, ensure there is the appropriate water pressure, and check for a blocked water port. If using a system such as Cavitron, the handpiece needs to be filled with water and the O-ring lubricated with water prior to placing the insert.

If a patient has a pacemaker, it is best to avoid use of magnetostrictive devices unless cleared by a medical professional. Piezoelectric devices are usually fine to use on a patient with a pacemaker. If you're ever unsure, always check with the patient's cardiologist.

Hand instrumentation

Understanding the various parts of a hand instrument will help you to determine where to use it and how.

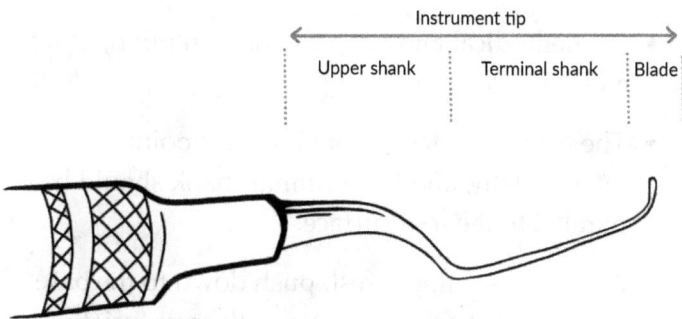

The various parts of the hand instrument tip

- **Angulation of the shank:** If the shank is straight, then that instrument should be used anteriorly; if the shank is more curved, that means it's for posterior teeth.

- **Tip of the blade:** If it's got a sharp end, it should be used supragingivally; if there is a blunt-ended blade, it should be used subgingivally.

- **Number of sharp edges:** If the blade has only one sharp edge, it's a Gracey, and you should only use that sharp side against the root surface. If both edges are sharp, then it is universal, and the instrument can be used on both sides.

- **Size of the blade:** If the blade is small, this is a mini curette, which is great for tight interproximal spaces, furcations, and the MINST approach. If it's a regular-sized blade, then that's a normal scaler.

Top tips on hand instrumentation:

- Be methodical and keep anatomy in mind, as it is a blind procedure.

- The tip of the blade should always point interdentally, and the terminal shank should be parallel to the root surface.

- Always use a finger rest, push down to the base of the pocket and scrape up with appropriate pressure against the root surface.

- Use a cotton roll/thin aspirator tip to collect the deposits.

Hand instruments that do not require sharpening are ideal; otherwise, it's important to ensure instruments are regularly and correctly sharpened at the practice or sent off to an external sharpening service.

Other

Other devices on the market can be very helpful in bio-film disruption as well as stain removal. AIRFLOW® by EMS is a popular option. Patients tend to accustom well to AIRFLOW and it can reduce the time required for treatment or SPC. It can be used prior to and after ultrasonic/hand instrumentation. The PLUS® powder can be used in all areas so would be the powder of choice when managing periodontitis patients. The PLUS powder is erythritol based (antibacterial component) and also contains chlorhexidine. This powder is suitable for all patients, including diabetics and vegans. Alternatively, the CLASSIC® powder would be limited to heavy stain removal on enamel.

There are many benefits of using EMS AIRFLOW with the PLUS powder:

1. Use of AIRFLOW at the start of treatment makes the calculus more visible.

2. At the end of treatment, it's great for stain removal and can access areas rubber cups will struggle to reach.

3. Excellent for orthodontic patients where access is difficult.

4. It's comfortable for patients.

5. Minimally invasive so less risk of damaging the tooth / root surface.

6. You can use it on soft tissue, for example the tongue if the patient has a tongue coating.

7. It can be used safely around implants.

When using the AIRFLOW, ensure the saliva ejector is at the back of the mouth and the high-volume suction is following the handpiece around the mouth. The AIRFLOW handpiece should not be used perpendicular to the tooth surface; keep it at a 3–5 mm distance and ensure continuous movement.

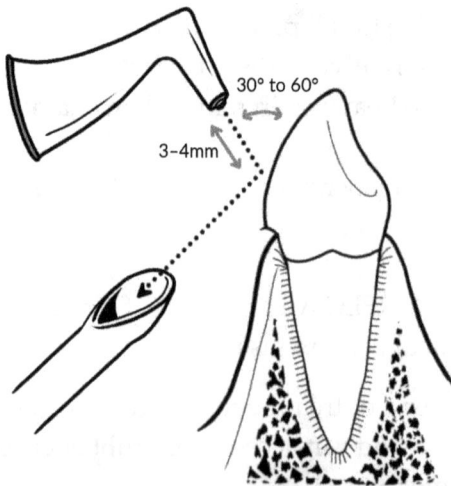

Position of the AIRFLOW and high-volume suction

In terms of settings, always keep the water on 100% and adjust the power as needed. There are a variety of other similar devices available.

9.7 RSI and back/neck pain

Non-surgical periodontal therapy can be taxing on the hands, wrists, and fingers, as well as the back, neck, and shoulders. As such, repetitive strain injury (RSI) is not uncommon among dentists. To reduce the chances of this, build in short rest periods, stretch and exercise your fingers while reaching for your next instrument, and build strength through the use of hand/grip-strengthening devices.

Ensure you think about your positioning as well as the use of loupes to reduce back/neck pain related to administering periodontal therapy.

10
Periodontal Challenges

There are a number of key challenges that we face when it comes to periodontal management. Occlusion is relevant to all forms of dentistry including periodontics, but is a topic of ongoing debate. Splinting is also a common treatment modality that is considered by dentists, but it's important to be aware of the indications and best ways of splinting. Furcations can be challenging to diagnose and manage. Then we have conditions such as dentine hypersensitivity and halitosis that are common in our periodontal patients yet may not always be straightforward to treat.

10.1 Occlusal trauma and splinting

Let's first turn our attention to occlusal trauma and indications for splinting.

Occlusal trauma

Traumatic occlusal force can be defined as 'any occlusal force resulting in injury to the teeth and/or the periodontal attachment apparatus' (Jepsen, 2018). Occlusal trauma is a term used to describe the injury to the periodontal attachment apparatus. A diagnosis may be made in the presence of one or more of the following: progressive tooth mobility, adaptive tooth mobility (fremitus), radiographically widened periodontal ligament space, tooth migration, discomfort/pain on chewing, and root resorption (Fan and Caton, 2018).

Primary occlusal trauma refers to damage that causes changes in the tissue due to excessive occlusal forces on a tooth or teeth that have healthy periodontal support (Jepsen, 2018). This type of trauma is characterised by adaptive mobility of the affected teeth and does not worsen over time. On the other hand, secondary occlusal trauma occurs when normal or excessive occlusal forces impact a tooth or teeth that have weakened periodontal support, such as in individuals with periodontitis (Jepsen, 2018). In cases of secondary trauma, teeth may show progressive mobility, migration, and discomfort during use.

Occlusal trauma is a co-factor that might increase the rate of progression of periodontitis (Passanezi and Sant'Ana, 2019). When treating patients with secondary occlusal trauma, the treatment of the periodontitis itself should remain the primary focus. In addition, if the patient has parafunctional habits, the provision of an occlusal splint should be considered. If occlusal adjustments are indicated to help correct occlusal disharmonies, these must be carried out carefully to preserve centric stops.

Splinting

The list below gives the key indications for permanent splinting (Hirschfield, 1937; Ferencz, 1987; Nyman and Lang, 1994):

- To immobilise mobile teeth that are causing discomfort or affecting function

- To immobilise teeth where there is progressive increase in mobility

- To prevent further movement of teeth, including drifting, overeruption, or relapse of orthodontically treated teeth

Temporary splinting is commonly used prior to completing treatment including regenerative therapy, and there is evidence to show that this will improve periodontal outcomes by reducing tooth mobility (Cortellini et al, 2001).

The periodontitis must be addressed prior to splinting, as a splint will make biofilm control more difficult. A range of different materials have been suggested and are used for splinting. One of the most common is a composite resin. However, composite resin alone is weak and brittle, so will fracture easily. Fibreglass-reinforced composite or archwire and composite would be more appropriate options. The latter is preferable whenever possible, as it allows some independent tooth movement, thus stimulating the periodontal ligament and alveolar bone, preventing atrophy. The use of fibre-reinforced composite resin produces a more rigid splint that can result in alveolar bone atrophy and may ultimately lead to the need to extract the tooth.

10.2 Furcations

A furcation defect can be defined as bone resorption and interradicular attachment loss in multirooted teeth (AAP, 2001). The assessment and classification of furcations was discussed in Chapter

3. Furcation involvement is more likely to occur in moderate-advanced periodontitis. In teeth with short root trunks, furcation involvement can occur earlier in disease. Maxillary molars are the most difficult to assess and treat as they have furcations with many entrances in the proximal areas. When assessing molar teeth from first to third, keep in mind that as you move further down the series:

- The roots become progressively shorter

- The roots divide more apically

- Access becomes more difficult for both the patient and clinician

- The space between the roots gets smaller

- The buccal plate gets thicker

- The prognosis gets poorer and the complexity of treatment becomes greater

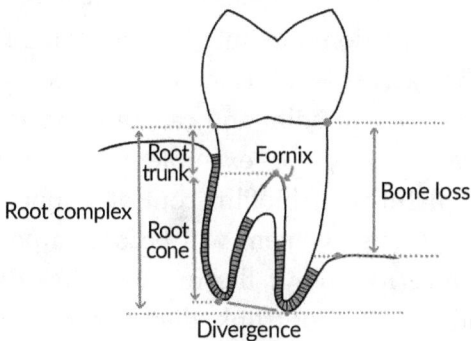

The components of the root complex and furcation area

Management of furcations

Teeth with furcation involvement due to periodontitis usually show progression if left untreated. The overall aims of treatment should be to eliminate/disrupt biofilm from the exposed surfaces of the root complex and to establish anatomy that facilitates self-performed biofilm control.

Summary of the treatment options available for furcations

Grade	Treatment options
I	Non-surgical treatment
II	Interproximal bone level below furcation entrance: furcation-plasty, apically positioned flap, tunnel prep, root resection/hemisection
	Interproximal bone level coronal to furcation entrance: regenerative therapy
III	Apically positioned flap, tunnel prep, root resection/hemisection, extraction

Biofilm control by non-surgical management (oral hygiene instruction and subgingival PMPR) is indicated when access is sufficient for brushes and instruments to control biofilm and calculus and to resolve any inflammation, for example Grade I FI buccal/lingual furca. If biofilm control is not optimal, non-surgical management will become a permanent maintenance routine. If the furcation has divergent roots and a short root trunk, then non-surgical treatment may be enough. In a Grade II or III furcation lesion it is almost impossible to render the lesion free of biofilm via conservative means.

Surgery may be used with either a resective or regenerative approach. For regenerative therapy, the procedures with the highest success for horizontal bone level gain are bone replacement grafts, guided tissue regeneration with resorbable membrane, plus bone replacement grafts and enamel matrix derivative (Jepsen et al, 2020).

Furcation-plasty involves both:

- **Odontoplasty:** Removal of tooth substance at the entrance of the furcation to eliminate or reduce the horizontal component of the defect. This aims to widen the entrance of the furcation and, therefore, improves the patient's ability to keep it clean. This can result in sensitivity, as the pulp is in close vicinity.

- **Osteoplasty:** Recontouring of the alveolar bone crest at the level of the furcation entrance. The aim is to reduce the buccolingual dimension of the bone crest in the furcation area.

Furcation-plasty is mainly used in buccal and lingual furca, as proximal sites are very difficult to access. However, if teeth are missing on either side of the tooth being treated, then access may be easier.

Tunnel preparation is often used as an adjunct to flap surgery for deep defects, and is more suitable for molars with short root trunks and wide divergent roots. The flap is raised, granulation tissue removed, root surfaces debrided, and interradicular bone removed.

Odontoplasty and osteoplasty may also be carried out. Flaps are then repositioned apically. The creation of a tunnel should facilitate cleaning with an interdental brush or similar. CHX and fluoride varnish might then be applied.

Root resection involves sectioning and removal of one or two of the roots of a multirooted tooth. All of the crown is retained. This is a good option if a couple of roots have suffered more bone loss, but the root to be retained has sufficient support. The tooth requires endodontic treatment prior to resection, and it is important not to leave behind a spur/projection following resection. Repreparation of what's left into a cleansable structure is often the key to success. It is usually advisable to place a crown following root resection.

Hemisection is the removal of a root and part of the crown that it supports. Again, this will first require endodontic treatment and a crown after treatment. This is often a good option for bruxists or if there is any type of occlusal trauma.

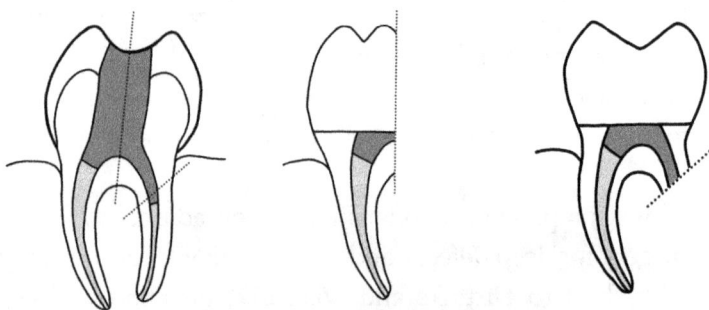

Hemisection vs root resection

Treatment may not always be possible, in which case extraction is an option. This might be considered when attachment loss is so great that none of the roots can be maintained; it could also be an option when treatment does not result in tooth/gingival anatomy that allows adequate self-performed oral hygiene. Extraction is also likely to be considered when a tooth has poor restorative/endodontic status, or when there is increased mobility; repeated periodontal abscesses; small, fused roots; and no strategic or aesthetic value to the tooth.

When considering the above treatment options, there are a number of tooth- and patient-related factors that need to be taken into account (Hughes, 2013).

Tooth-related factors:

- **Root trunk length:** Generally, shorter root trunks are preferable. Early furcation involvement in disease means remaining periodontal tissues are more likely to support the roots. Longer root trunks indicate advanced furcation involvement with reduced support for stability.

- **Root cone divergence:** Smaller divergence complicates access and separation. Orthodontic treatment can increase the distance between roots after separation, aiding in cleaning and restoration.

- **Length and shape of root cones:** Short and small roots are less stable after separation. Thin roots with narrow canals pose endodontic treatment challenges. Small roots are also inadequate as abutments for prosthetic procedures.

- **Fusion of root cones:** Separation is technically challenging. Fusion can be identified through clinical assessment, radiographs, and flap surgery.

- **Remaining support around individual roots:** This is determined by probing around the separated roots. Minimal remaining support makes the root a poor candidate for restorative treatment and less likely to be stable.

- **Stability of individual roots:** Assess stability after separation.

- **Access for oral hygiene aids:** Post-treatment, the tooth must allow for effective oral hygiene. If not, long-term treatment success is compromised.

Patient-related factors include:

- Patient opinion
- Smoker – one would likely avoid any surgical treatment
- Cost
- Predictability
- General health and age

- Functional and aesthetic demands
- Level of biofilm control
- Access

10.3 Dentine hypersensitivity

Dentine hypersensitivity (DH) is 'characterised by a short, sharp pain arising from exposed dentine in response to stimuli – typically thermal, evaporative, tactile, osmotic, or chemical – that cannot be ascribed to any other form of dental defect or pathology' (Holland et al, 1997). A practice-based study of 18–35-year-olds found an incidence rate for DH of 42% (West et al, 2013).

The aetiology of DH can be attributed to Brannstrom's hydrodynamic theory, which describes the fluid movement within the dentinal tubules. For DH to occur, there must be (West et al, 2015):

1. Dentine exposure (lesion localisation) – soft tissue loss (gingival recession) or hard tissue loss (abrasion and erosion)

2. Tubule exposure (lesion initiation) – abrasion or erosion

Dentine hypersensitivity is not uncommon amongst periodontitis patients, and it can also present following periodontal treatment. It is distressing and can affect the patient's quality of life.

Management of DH

The first steps in management are to modify or eliminate the aetiological and predisposing factors. This might include:

- Appropriate home care regime

- Treatment of periodontitis

- Dietary advice

- Referral to the GP if there are any signs of reflux

- Mouthguard if there are any signs of parafunction

The next step would be to recommend the use of proven, efficacious products that are available over the counter, such as toothpaste or tooth mousse. Professionally applied agents would be reserved for the more severe or non-responding cases (West et al, 2015). In terms of the evidence base, there is sound evidence for the use of products containing: stannous fluoride, strontium acetate, arginine/calcium carbonate, and/or calcium sodium phosphosilicate (West et al, 2015). If this doesn't work, you can move on to professionally applied products, including varnish and dentine adhesive sealers. In terms of their mode of action, agents may cause nerve desensitisation or tubule occlusion.

When treating patients with DH either during active treatment or SPC, ensure they are as comfortable as possible by rubbing prophy polish onto the tooth, using ultrasonics with warm water and, if needed, giving local anaesthesia.

10.4 Halitosis

Halitosis (from the Latin for breath, *halitus*, and the Greek suffix *osis*, meaning abnormal) is the presence of unpleasant or offensive breath odour independent of its origin (Greenman et al, 2005). Halitosis can have significant detrimental social implications for the sufferer and can have a significant impact on their normal social interactions (Eli et al, 2001).

The exact prevalence of halitosis remains unclear. Many epidemiological studies are challenging to assess since they often rely on subjective self-reports of bad breath, which tend to lack accuracy and sensitivity. Nevertheless, existing data indicates that halitosis is a widespread issue that can impact individuals across various age groups. Most research suggests that around 30% of the population experiences halitosis (van Dortsten and Van der Weijden, 2007).

Intra-oral halitosis, often referred to as oral malodour, pertains to cases where the cause of bad breath originates within the oral cavity. By contrast, extra-oral halitosis arises from sources outside the mouth, which can be categorised into blood-borne and non-blood-borne types. Additionally, conditions such as pseudo-halitosis and halitophobia describe individuals who believe they have halitosis despite professional evaluations indicating otherwise. Other forms of halitosis include temporary or transient halitosis, as well as 'morning breath'.

Research indicates that approximately 85% of individuals with persistent genuine halitosis have odours originating from inside the mouth (Scully et al, 2001). The primary cause of intra-oral halitosis is often attributed to tongue coating, while gingivitis and periodontitis can also contribute to the condition. Various acute conditions, including peri-coronal infections, acute herpetic gingivostomatitis, and necrotising gingivitis, can produce a notably strong odour known as 'foetor oris'. Additionally, factors such as xerostomia (dry mouth), oral candidiasis, certain medications, poorly fitting restorations, and dental caries may further exacerbate intra-oral halitosis (Kumar et al, 2014).

Intra-oral halitosis is primarily caused by the release of volatile compounds resulting from bacterial degradation of epithelial cells, salivary and serum proteins, and food residues. Numerous molecular species can contribute to the overall malodour, though key among those are volatile sulphur compounds such as methyl mercaptan, hydrogen sulphide, and dimethyl sulphide. The formation of these compounds occurs through the breakdown of organic debris and protein substrates by various anaerobic bacteria, particularly those with proteolytic capabilities (Miller and Dyer, 2011).

The dorsum of the tongue serves as an ideal habitat for anaerobic bacteria, due to the favourable redox potential found in the deep crypts associated with the structure of the tongue papillae. The tongue coating consists of shed epithelial cells, food particles, bacteria, and salivary proteins, creating an environment conducive to producing volatile sulphur compounds and other odorous substances (Roldán et al, 2013). Anaerobic bacteria also play a crucial role in the subgingival plaque associated with periodontitis, where elevated levels of volatile sulphur compounds are often detected in periodontal pockets and gingival crevicular fluid from individuals suffering from gingivitis or periodontitis (Scully et al, 2001).

To diagnose halitosis, a comprehensive approach is necessary, including a detailed medical history, examination of soft tissues for tongue coating, periodontal assessment, and an organoleptic evaluation. During the organoleptic assessment, the clinician evaluates the odour of exhaled air from both the mouth and nose. At the most basic level, clinicians can use their own judgement to determine the presence or absence of malodour in a patient (Yoshida et al, 2014).

Management of halitosis

The treatment of halitosis is primarily determined by its underlying cause. Once intra-oral halitosis has been diagnosed, you should sensitively let the patient know about their diagnosis but keep the conversation focused on how we can help them address this. For management, you should take the following steps:

1. Provide personalised guidance on halitosis, discussing the specific causes that are relevant to the patient. Highlight the importance of self-care practices to improve the condition, and reassure the patient that effective treatment can help reduce or eliminate bad breath (Friedman et al, 2015).

2. Encourage the patient to refrain from smoking and limit the intake of foods that may contribute to halitosis.

3. Advise the patient to maintain oral moisture by staying hydrated and using sugar-free chewing gum to stimulate saliva production (Scully et al, 2001).

4. Optimise the patient's oral hygiene routine by recommending brushing teeth twice daily and incorporating daily interdental cleaning to remove biofilm and food particles (Sanz et al, 2015).

5. Instruct and motivate the patient to use a tongue scraper if tongue coating is present, as tongue cleaning has been shown to be an effective method for reducing intra-oral halitosis caused by bacteria on the tongue (Roldán et al, 2013; Outhouse et al, 2006).

6. Suggest the use of chemical agents with proven efficacy if necessary (Slot et al, 2015). Mouth rinses and toothpaste containing active ingredients like chlorhexidine, cetylpyridinium chloride, and zinc compounds (such as CHX+CPC+Zn and ZnCl+CPC) can help to significantly reduce halitosis (Rosenberg et al, 2006).

7. Provide periodontal treatment if the patient exhibits signs of gingivitis or periodontitis. Additionally, address any other oral health issues that may contribute to halitosis.

8. Identify and rectify local dental factors such as overhanging restorations and dental caries that may exacerbate the condition.

9. Review the patient's halitosis status after appropriate therapy, suggesting further measures if the issue persists.

It is crucial to recognise that a small percentage of patients, less than 10%, may suffer from extra-oral halitosis or halitophobia and might need to be referred to a medical specialist. This could include consultations with oral medicine specialists, otorhinolaryngologists, to check for chronic tonsillitis or sinusitis, or physicians to assess potential underlying conditions such as gastrointestinal, hepatic, endocrine, pulmonary, or renal diseases. Referral to a psychologist or psychiatrist may also be necessary for those experiencing halitophobia (Yoshida et al, 2014).

11
Periodontal Emergencies And Their Management

P atients might often present to us in pain or with acute problems that cause them to seek urgent care. It's important to be aware of these 'periodontal emergencies' and be confident in solving them efficiently. In this chapter, we will cover a range of conditions that may present as an emergency.

11.1 Gingival abscess

A gingival abscess is 'a localised purulent infection affecting the marginal gingiva or interdental papillae' (AAP, 2000). Clinically, it is characterised by a rapidly expanding localised swelling, which may present as either shiny and smooth or pointed. The presence of suppuration is common, and patients often experience significant pain and tenderness upon palpation of the affected area.

Gingival abscesses frequently occur due to the impaction of subgingival foreign objects and typically develop in previously healthy gingivae. The literature implicates various foreign bodies, such as fragments of nails in individuals with nail-biting habits. For abscesses caused by the impaction of oral hygiene aids, the term 'oral hygiene abscesses' has been suggested (Gillette, 1980).

Management of a gingival abscess involves incision, drainage, and irrigation with saline to alleviate acute symptoms. Addressing the underlying cause is crucial, and mechanical debridement may be beneficial in this regard. The short-term use of chlorhexidine mouthwash or warm saline rinses is commonly recommended, particularly when the area is too tender for brushing. Follow-up appointments are necessary to ensure resolution.

11.2 Periodontal abscess

A periodontal abscess is defined as a localised buildup of pus within the gingival wall of a periodontal pocket, resulting in the destruction of collagen fibre attachment and the loss of nearby alveolar bone. Clinically, it often appears as an ovoid swelling on the lateral side of the tooth root. In some cases, abscesses that are deeper within the periodontium may show up as diffuse swelling or reddening, with the affected area typically being sensitive to touch. This condition is usually associated with a deep periodontal pocket and may cause bleeding and discomfort when probing. Suppuration might occur through a fistula or an opening in the periodontal pocket, which could be spontaneous or triggered by finger pressure (Herrera et al, 2000).

Common signs of a periodontal abscess include increased tooth mobility and tenderness on percussion, and the patient might report that the tooth feels 'high in their bite'. Radiographs often reveal some degree of bone loss around the affected tooth, and sensibility testing should provide a positive response.

A periodontal abscess is often a complication of existing periodontitis, especially in cases with complex morphology, furcation involvement, or vertical defects, where the closure of the pocket margins can lead to infection spreading to adjacent periodontal tissues. Factors such as changes in the subgingival microbiota, increased bacterial virulence, or reduced host defences can impair the drainage of pus, leading to the development of an abscess. This can occur in situations such as:

- Following subgingival PMPR, where calculus fragments may become dislodged and pushed into the periodontal tissues (Dello Russo, 1985).

- After surgical therapy, associated with foreign bodies like membranes or sutures (Garrett et al, 1997).

- Acute exacerbation of periodontitis (Fine, 1994).

- Systemic antimicrobial intake without subgingival debridement in severe periodontitis, leading to overgrowth of opportunistic bacteria (Helovuo et al, 1993).

Managing a periodontal abscess involves addressing the acute symptoms to prevent further tissue damage. If the tooth can be saved, the first step is to establish drainage either through the periodontal pocket or via an external incision, followed by thorough cleaning of the area. Adjusting the occlusion can offer immediate relief. Systemic antibiotics are only necessary if there is systemic involvement or if the infection is spreading.

If the tooth is deemed unsalvageable, extraction may be the most appropriate course of action. Since most periodontal abscesses occur in areas with pre-existing periodontal issues, it is crucial to reassess periodontal treatment once the acute phase has resolved. For patients who have not previously received treatment, appropriate periodontal care should be initiated. For those already undergoing treatment, it should continue after addressing the acute abscess. For patients receiving supportive periodontal therapy, any potential recurrence of the abscess should be carefully evaluated, including assessing the extent of tissue damage and its effect on the tooth's long-term prognosis (Herrera, 2000).

11.3 Pericoronitis/peri-coronal abscess

Pericoronitis is the inflammation of the soft tissues surrounding the crown of a partially erupted tooth, whereas a peri-coronal abscess refers to the localised accumulation of pus within the gingival flap overlying an incompletely erupted tooth. The condition most frequently affects the partially erupted and impacted mandibular third molar, as the overlying operculum provides a perfect environment for debris and bacteria accumulation. Trauma from an opposing tooth often exacerbates the condition.

Clinically, patients often present with a red, swollen, and potentially suppurative lesion that is painful to touch. Common symptoms include cheek swelling at the mandibular angle, trismus, and radiating pain to the ear. Systemic complications such as lymphadenopathy, fever, and general malaise may also occur.

In terms of management, after administering anaesthesia, the operculum should be irrigated to remove debris. In some instances, you might need to excise the operculum and carry out occlusal adjustment on the opposing tooth to prevent further trauma. Antibiotics are recommended only if there are systemic symptoms or evidence of spreading infection. Once the acute infection phase has resolved, you must decide whether there is any need for tooth extraction.

11.4 Necrotising gingivitis and periodontitis

Necrotising periodontal diseases are among the most severe inflammatory lesions linked to the oral biofilm; they commonly affect the mandibular anterior teeth. Necrotising gingivitis is marked by necrosis and ulcers in the free gingiva, often starting at the interdental papilla and presenting a 'punched-out' appearance. Marginal erythema and progression to the marginal gingiva may occur, with a pseudo-membrane forming over the necrotic area. Removing this pseudo-membrane reveals underlying connective tissue that bleeds. Pain severity correlates with the extent of the lesion and typically increases with eating and oral hygiene activities. Additional symptoms may include halitosis, fever, and malaise.

Necrotising periodontitis shares these features but also involves necrosis of the periodontal ligament and alveolar bone, causing attachment loss. Disease progression can result in an interproximal crater separating the buccal and lingual/palatal parts of the papilla. Deep craters may denude the interdental crestal bone, and lateral spread of interproximal necrosis can create extensive destruction zones. Severe cases can involve bone sequestration. Associated risk factors include high stress, heavy smoking, and poor nutrition. Both necrotising gingivitis and periodontitis may be linked to untreated HIV/AIDS, other immunocompromising conditions, or immunosuppressive drugs.

Treatment of both conditions involves careful superficial debridement to remove biofilm and calculus, preferably using ultrasonic instruments to minimise pressure on ulcerated tissues. Debridement should be done daily and progressively deeper as patient tolerance improves, typically over two to four days during the acute phase. To reduce pain and aid healing, mechanical oral hygiene should be limited, and patients should use chemical plaque control agents like 0.2% chlorhexidine mouthwash twice daily. Additional antibacterial effects against anaerobes can be achieved with 3% hydrogen peroxide diluted 1:1 with warm water or other oxygen-releasing agents. If periodontal condition does not improve with debridement alone, systemic antimicrobials, such as metronidazole (400 mg TDS for five days), should be considered due to their efficacy against strict anaerobes (Loesche et al, 1982).

As symptoms and signs improve, strict oral hygiene should be enforced and debridement completed as necessary. The post-acute phase of management should address any pre-existing periodontal disease and systemic risk factors, with close monitoring and support for affected patients.

11.5 Acute herpetic gingivostomatitis

Herpetic gingivostomatitis is a prevalent viral infection of the oral mucosa, characterised by small ulcers with raised edges. These ulcers can appear across various areas in the mouth, including both attached and unattached mucosal surfaces. Caused by the herpes simplex virus, herpetic gingivostomatitis is the initial manifestation of primary herpes simplex infection, which is more severe than subsequent presentations such as herpes labialis. Patients often experience generalised pain in the gingiva and oral mucosa, along with systemic symptoms like lymphadenopathy, fever, and malaise. The lesions typically persist for seven to ten days and heal without leaving scars. This condition is most frequently observed in children aged two to five years.

Given that the condition is self-limiting, treatment primarily focuses on hydration and symptom management. Palliative care is important to relieve pain and ensure the patient can eat and drink. Paracetamol is commonly administered, with the recommended dosage for children aged two to four years being 180 mg every four to six hours. In severe cases, especially in immunocompromised patients, hospital referral is necessary for potential intravenous antiviral treatment.

11.6 Acute physical/ chemical/thermal injury

This category of acute periodontal lesions is not caused by the oral biofilm but understanding these conditions is crucial for accurate diagnosis and effective treatment.

Physical injuries may present as erosions or ulcers, sometimes accompanied by gingival recession. Less commonly, they can manifest as hyperkeratosis, vesicles, or bullae. Continuous mild trauma might lead to hyperkeratotic lesions, while more aggressive trauma can cause superficial lacerations. These injuries can be either asymptomatic or cause intense localised pain.

Physical injuries to the oral tissues can often stem from poor oral hygiene practices, trauma, or parafunctional habits. For example, using a harsh toothpaste and brushing too aggressively can lead to gingival ulcers or erosions. Similarly, improper use of dental floss or other interdental tools may cause gingival ulceration, inflammation, and recession. In children and teenagers, self-inflicted injuries are common and can involve fingers, nails, or objects like pencils (Creath et al, 1995; Krejci, 2000). Traumatic injuries can also result from broken teeth, orthodontic appliances, or oral piercings.

Thermal injuries are typically painful, with gingival tissues appearing erythematous and desquamated, sometimes accompanied by vesicles, erosions, or ulcers. Such injuries are often caused by burns from hot food or drinks.

Chemical lesions occur after direct contact with a chemical agent on the mucosa, resulting in maculae, vesicles, erosions, or ulcers, depending on the agent and duration of exposure (Herrera et al, 2014). Common sources include oral bleaching agents, etchants, and certain dental products, especially when used improperly or with ill-fitting trays (Sapir and Bimstein, 2000; De Bruyne et al, 2000).

Treatment of the above depends on the diagnosis and the source of trauma, so a thorough clinical examination and patient history are essential to identify the cause. Management involves eliminating the initiating factor and addressing pain symptoms. Generally, lesions heal without further intervention, but additional treatment may sometimes be necessary. It is important to differentiate these lesions from those associated with mucocutaneous diseases, which may not have a clear initiating factor. In such cases, mechanical oral hygiene may be paused, and chemical plaque control can be used to help identify the cause.

11.7 Subgingival root fractures

When a tooth fracture extends from the supragingival area apically in a subgingival direction, it can cause acute pain and lead to periodontal infection. Patients may or may not recall a specific traumatic event during chewing. Key risk factors include heavily restored teeth without cuspal coverage and those with bruxism. Additionally, fractures are common in patients with reduced periodontium due to an unfavourable crown-to-root ratio.

Magnification and good lighting are essential for identifying fracture lines. Diagnostic tools such as a 'tooth sleuth' can help by applying occlusal pressure to individual cusps. Even if a fracture line is not visible, fractured teeth often present with a localised deep pocket depth and potentially an abscess. The affected tooth or fractured cusp might be highly sensitive to percussion or may only cause pain upon release of biting pressure. Fractures can be vertical along the root axis or angled, with varying degrees of root involvement.

Management of tooth fractures depends on the vitality of the tooth and the fracture's location and extent. Initial steps might involve removing existing restorations to thoroughly assess the tooth and confirm the diagnosis. Treatment options typically include endodontic therapy followed by a full coverage restoration if the tooth can be saved. A periodontal flap can be helpful for better visualisation of the fracture, and crown lengthening might be necessary to expose the most apical part of the fracture. If the tooth is deemed untreatable, extraction will be required.

12
Supportive Periodontal Care

Supportive periodontal care (SPC) is an effective and integral component of managing periodontitis patients. Its importance should be emphasised to patients before commencing any active treatment. With supportive periodontal therapy, periodontal health can be maintained in most patients, even in advanced cases (Rosling et al, 2001).

The aims of SPC are to:

- Monitor whether the condition is stable and provide an opportunity to initiate treatment if progression is detected

- Remove aetiological factors before the disease progresses

- Reinforce smoking cessation and organise referral if appropriate

12.1 Recall interval

Recall intervals should be determined based on the patient's risk profile. The default is usually three months but can be up to twelve months. The recall interval needs to be reviewed at every visit and if needed adjusted. When considering risk and tailoring the recall interval, there are several patient, treatment, and local factors to consider.

Patient factors

Patients with periodontitis who smoke are more prone to the disease and generally experience less favourable treatment outcomes (Tomar and Asma, 2000). This necessitates more frequent dental appointments for monitoring and management (Heasman et al, 2006). Similarly, systemic conditions like uncontrolled diabetes significantly increase the likelihood of periodontitis recurrence, thus requiring patients to have more regular check-ups (Löe, 1993). High stress levels in patients can also warrant more frequent maintenance visits to manage periodontal health effectively (Genco et al, 1999).

Advancements in genetic research have identified markers that help determine a patient's susceptibility to periodontal diseases. Notably, studies on interleukin-1 (IL-1) polymorphisms reveal that patients with IL-1 genotype positivity are more likely to suffer from advanced periodontitis and see higher rates of tooth loss (Kornman et al, 1997). Additionally, patients classified as high risk (Grade C) due to previous susceptibility to severe periodontitis will also need more frequent reassessment and follow-up appointments to manage their condition effectively.

Previous treatment

The interval is also dependent on previous treatment. For example, if there has been recent surgery, the patient will have to be seen sooner than for non-surgical treatment. The outcome of active treatment needs to be considered too, as the limitations of active treatment are likely to continue during maintenance, and this may warrant a shorter recall interval.

Local factors

Since biofilm is by far the most important aetiologic agent for the occurrence of periodontal diseases, the full-mouth assessment of the bacterial load is critical in the determination of the risk of disease recurrence. In general, inadequate biofilm management will necessitate more frequent dental visits. However, the amount of biofilm that can be maintained without disease progression can differ from patient to patient. For those facing challenges with biofilm control – whether due to overcrowded or misaligned teeth, or physical limitations – more frequent assistance may be essential.

The type of periodontal disease present, such as infrabony lesions, furcation involvement, or gum recession, is also significant. Multi-rooted teeth are particularly vulnerable to loss during the maintenance phase (Mavridis and Mavridis, 2018). Additionally, the presence of root grooves and concavities can further elevate the risk of recurrence, indicating a need for more regular maintenance visits.

When considering the severity of past or existing periodontal disease, factors such as age-related bone loss, tooth loss, BoP, and the depth of pockets (5 mm or deeper) are important. The absence of BoP is a strong indicator of periodontal stability, while a high prevalence of deep residual pockets during SPC suggests an increased likelihood of disease progression (Trombelli et al, 2015).

Patients with concurrent oral conditions, like erosive lichen planus or mucous membrane pemphigoid, may also require more frequent appointments, as their symptoms can make plaque control more challenging.

Various tools are now available to assist in determining periodontal risk that can help with the above considerations, and in general risk assessment for our patients. For example, PreViser / DEPPA technology is an online assessment tool that evaluates eleven factors: patient age, smoking, diabetes, history of periodontal surgery, pocket depth, BoP, furcation involvements, subgingival restorations, root calculus, radiographic bone height, and the presence of vertical bone lesions (Meyer and Lewis, 2018). A patient report is then produced as a biofeedback and communication tool.

The Periodontal Risk Assessment (PRA) is another online tool that has been widely used in specialist teaching programmes (Cortellini and Tonetti, 2005). It is often referred to as the 'spider diagram', as it produces a functional graphical representation of a patient's risk based on six clinical, systemic, and environmental factors: percentage bleeding on probing, number of residual periodontal pockets ≥5 mm, number of lost teeth, alveolar bone loss in relation to patient age, systemic and/or genetic predispositions, and environmental factors (such as tobacco use). This then guides the recall interval.

12.2 Palliative periodontal care

In the ideal scenario, there would be no (or very few) periodontal probing depths of 4 mm with bleeding or 5 mm and above when a patient enters SPC. However, in the case that a patient moves to supportive care with acceptance of deep pockets, this is termed palliative periodontal care.

The aim here is to slow down the progression of the condition, though active treatment is not occurring; in other words, the condition will not improve. Palliative periodontal care may be needed when risk factors remain unchanged. For example, if the patient is a smoker and not keen to stop, then after two rounds of active treatment, you would not continue to repeat this. Or if the patient's biofilm self-care does not improve and you've persisted with numerous efforts, you may wish to place them on palliative care until this changes.

Patients can move back into the active treatment phase if these factors change, for instance, if the patient stops smoking or the biofilm control improves. Sometimes, pockets may be accepted when, for example, the patient has declined a referral, and you do not feel you can achieve much more improvement.

12.3 Appointment structure

The content of the SPC appointment depends on the type of treatment completed and the outcome. A typical visit after successful non-surgical treatment would involve:

1. Checking the patient's medical history

2. Reviewing their oral hygiene regime and revising if necessary

3. Reviewing and discussing control of any other risk factors

4. Probing all sites to check probing depth and bleeding after probing – a full six-point pocket chart is required on a yearly basis

5. Supragingival PMPR as needed

Supportive periodontal care after partially successful non-surgical treatment – ie some residual deep pockets and inflammation remain – will include all of the above steps plus as much subgingival PMPR of residual deep pockets as is practically possible.

There may be occasions where a significant relapse in the periodontal condition gives rise to the need for the patient to enter the active treatment phase. The patient may then require a few dedicated appointments for subgingival PMPR to get them back on track; they will then enter SPC again.

13
Dental Implants

Professor Brånemark is considered the pioneer of titanium endosseous dental implants. He presented ten years of research at Cambridge University showing that bone can grow intimately onto the surface of titanium implants, in a process known as osseointegration (Brånemark et al, 1977). This discovery paved the way for further development of dental applications.

Dental implants have become a common solution for replacing missing teeth. It's important for patients to understand that restorations supported by implants necessitate ongoing maintenance and can give rise to complications, such as peri-implantitis, which may impact the implant's success and lifespan. Dental professionals are responsible for evaluating the health of the tissues surrounding the implants and identifying any potential peri-implant complications.

IMPLANTS: KEY TERMINOLOGY

- **Osseointegration:** A direct structural and functional connection between ordered, living bone, and the surface of a load-carrying implant.

- **Endosseous dental implant:** A device inserted into the jawbone (endosseous) to support a dental prosthesis. It is the 'tooth root' analogue and is often referred to as a 'fixture'.

- **Implant abutment:** The component that attaches to the dental implant and supports the prosthesis. A transmucosal abutment is one that passes through the mucosa overlying the implant. A temporary or healing abutment may be used during the healing of the peri-implant soft tissue before the definitive abutment is chosen.

- **Abutment screw:** A screw used to connect an abutment to the implant.

- **Single-stage implant surgery:** Involves surgically placing a dental implant that is left exposed to the oral cavity following insertion. This protocol is used in non-submerged implant systems.

- **Two-stage implant surgery:** This involves the initial surgical placement of a dental implant, which is buried beneath the mucosa and then subsequently exposed with a second surgical procedure some months later. It is used in submerged implant systems.

There are notable distinctions between natural teeth and dental implants. The periodontal complex surrounding a tooth has evolved over millions of years and is made up of highly specialised tissues, whereas the soft tissue surrounding implants essentially consists of scar tissue. Osseointegration occurs as a reaction to the foreign material, leading to direct contact between bone and implant, accompanied by the formation of a soft-tissue scar. Given these differences, it is reasonable to conclude that the tissues around natural teeth and the peri-implant mucosa around implants will not function in the same manner.

The table below outlines the histological comparison of the periodontium versus peri-implant tissues (Jung and Ganeles, 2013):

Jung and Ganeles' (2013) comparison of periodontium and peri-implant tissues

Periodontium	Peri-implant mucosa
Anchoring system of root cementum, alveolar bone, and desmodontic fibres. Tooth not in direct contact with bone.	Direct bone-to-implant contact. No periodontal ligament or cementum.
More sub-epithelial fibroblasts and vessels. Increased vascularisation. Low collagen to fibroblast ratio.	More sub-epithelial collagen fibres and fewer fibroblasts. Reduced vascularisation. High collagen-to-fibroblast ratio.
Dento-gingival, dento-periosteal, circular, and trans-septal fibre orientation.	Parallel orientation of collagen fibres in relation to implant surface – fibres not inserted directly into implant.

Jung and Ganeles' (2013) comparison of periodontium and peri-implant tissues (cont)

Periodontium	Peri-implant mucosa
Junctional epithelium originated from reduced enamel epithelium. Basal lamina and hemi desmosomes. Complete attachment to enamel.	Junctional epithelium originates from oral epithelium: basal lamina and hemi desmosomes. Poorly adherent, poor regenerative capacity.

Compared to periodontal tissues, it is suggested that peri-implant tissues are more susceptible to inflammatory reactions, a phenomenon also confirmed immunohistochemically with an increase of inflammatory infiltrate in comparison with natural teeth (Nishihara et al, 2015).

13.1 Dental implants in periodontitis patients

There are several important factors to be aware of when considering periodontitis patients who have dental implants.

Risk of peri-implant disease

Patients with a history of periodontitis face an increased risk of developing peri-implantitis (Schwarz et al, 2011). Long-term studies indicate that these individuals tend to have greater probing depths and bone loss around implants, along with a higher occurrence of peri-implantitis and elevated overall failure rates (Roccuzzo et al, 2023). Research has shown that implants placed in patients with periodontal susceptibility experience significantly more bone loss than those placed in periodontally healthy individuals, regardless of the type of implant used (Lang et al, 2011). Therefore, it is crucial to address and manage periodontitis prior to implant placement, ensuring that any deep probing depths are resolved (Sgolastra et al, 2015). Additionally, individuals with a history of periodontitis should be informed during the consent process about their increased risk of complications associated with implant procedures.

Implant position

Implants should not be positioned too closely together, as this can hinder effective biofilm management. Whenever feasible, it is recommended to maintain a spacing of at least 3 mm between implants (Schwarz et al, 2015). Any historical loss of hard or soft tissues may affect the ability to position the implant correctly in three dimensions, so this must be considered prior to placing. Improper buccolingual positioning can result in restorations that have difficult-to-clean overhangs. Additionally, placing implants too deeply can lead to increased probing depths and a significant subgingival environment, which complicates optimal biofilm control. It's essential to consider these potential complications during the planning phase and to evaluate the need for bone and/or soft-tissue grafting when necessary.

Screw versus cement

Whenever possible, screw-retained restorations are recommended. When opting for cemented restorations, care must be taken to avoid excess cement from being extruded into the peri-implant sulcus during the seating process. Deeper crown margins typically lead to a higher volume of excess cement. Any leftover cement can create a rough surface that facilitates microbial colonisation, potentially resulting in peri-implant mucositis and even peri-implantitis (Salgado et al, 2016). Excess cement can also act as a foreign body, triggering an inflammatory response that may contribute to the development of peri-implantitis.

Removable options

It may not always be necessary to provide a fixed restoration. Overdentures are often a more easily cleaned and safer long-term solution for some patients (Zitzmann and Marinello, 2001). A removable prosthesis can replace both hard and soft tissue, which might provide a better aesthetic outcome as well as allow better access to the peri-implant tissues for ongoing plaque control.

The McGill consensus statement from 2002 (Feine et al, 2002) concludes that: 'patients are significantly more satisfied with implant supported overdentures compared to conventional overdentures. Patients experience more stable dentures, greater ease when chewing, greater comfort and can speak more easily.'

Supportive peri-implant care

Longitudinal studies have shown that a lack of supportive therapy is associated with a higher frequency of peri-implantitis (Sanz et al, 2015). For this reason, supportive peri-implant care is integral to minimising risks. Recall intervals should be tailored according to previous periodontal therapy, the location of the soft tissues, the implant location, and the prosthesis design (Pjetursson et al, 2012).

Extracting teeth to replace with implants

There is now a growing body of evidence to suggest that maintaining periodontally involved teeth can provide better tooth survival outcomes and can also be more cost-effective than placing implant-retained crowns (Kumar et al, 2015; Misch et al, 2014; Pjetursson and Lang, 2008). Thus, there has been a gradual move towards retaining periodontally involved teeth for as long as possible before replacement with implants.

13.2 Key recommendations

Below are the key recommendations from the European Federation of Periodontology (Herrera et al, 2022) with regard to dental implants:

- Patients must be made aware of the potential risks of biological complications, such as peri-implant diseases, and the importance of preventive care.

- A thorough and individual risk assessment should be conducted, taking into account both systemic and local risk factors. Modifiable risks, such as persistent probing pocket depth in the remaining teeth and smoking habits, should be addressed. As such, management of periodontal disease to eliminate residual pockets that bleed upon probing, along with smoking cessation, should occur before placing implants.

- It is crucial to ensure that implant components and the superstructure fit properly, in order to minimise areas where biofilm can accumulate. If cemented implant restorations are chosen, the margins of the restoration should align with the mucosal margin to facilitate the effective removal of excess cement.

- Placing implants at a submucosal level to conceal crown margins might increase the risk of peri-implant diseases.

- To enhance personal oral hygiene, clinicians should aim to have keratinised, attached, and stable tissue surrounding the transmucosal part of the implant during initial placement (for one-stage procedures) or during abutment connection (for two-stage procedures).

- Infection control is critical in preventing peri-implant diseases; therefore, patients should receive clear instructions regarding their oral hygiene practices, along with regular monitoring and reinforcement of these practices.

- The placement of the implant and the design of the prosthesis should allow for adequate access to facilitate regular diagnostic probing and both personal and professional oral hygiene.

- Professional supportive care for peri-implant health should be tailored to the specific needs of each patient, with recall intervals set at three, six, or twelve months, depending on their compliance. During these visits, peri-implant tissues should be carefully examined, including probing assessments, with a particular focus on any bleeding upon probing.

13.3 Management of peri-implant disease

In a healthy state, it's essential to reinforce self-care biofilm control through personalised oral hygiene instructions. In addition to using a manual or electric toothbrush, patients may be advised to incorporate interdental brushes, superfloss, single-tufted brushes, and possibly irrigation devices into their routine. Patients should also be enrolled in a supportive peri-implant care programme.

For cases of peri-implant mucositis, the focus of intervention is on effective biofilm control, which can be achieved through self-care or professional treatment. Outcomes should be assessed after a period of two to three months, and if peri-implant health has not been restored, re-treatment is recommended. Addressing peri-implant mucositis is crucial for preventing progression to peri-implantitis.

In instances of peri-implantitis, referral to a specialist or back to the original dental professional who placed the implant may be necessary. Various treatment strategies for peri-implantitis have been proposed, generally based on protocols used for periodontal disease in natural teeth. A Cochrane systematic review published in 2008 and updated in 2012 (Friedman, 2012), which included nine randomised controlled trials, concluded that 'there is no evidence to suggest a superior protocol for the management of peri-implantitis.' Proposed treatments encompass both non-surgical and surgical options, with or without adjunctive therapies. Typically, an initial non-surgical treatment phase, including submarginal instrumentation, is carried out. Following this, a re-evaluation of clinical outcomes will determine whether the patient should enter a secondary preventive supportive peri-implant care programme or proceed to surgical intervention, assuming the affected implant is still considered treatable (Herrera et al, 2022).

14
Multidisciplinary Care

Successful periodontal care often involves interaction with other specialties. In this chapter, we will focus on the perio–endo and the perio–ortho interfaces.

14.1 The perio-endo interface

According to the updated classification (Papapanou et al, 2018), an endo–perio lesion is a pathological communication between the pulpal and periodontal tissues of a given tooth, which occurs in either an acute or chronic form. These lesions can be further classified according to their signs and symptoms, which have a direct impact on their prognosis and treatment (eg presence or absence of fractures and perforations, and presence or absence of periodontitis).

Endo–perio lesions can be triggered by a carious or traumatic lesion that affects the pulp and, secondarily, the periodontium; by periodontal destruction that secondarily affects the root canal; or by the concomitant presence of both pathologies. There is no evidence for a distinct pathophysiology between an endo–periodontal and a periodontal lesion (Santos et al, 2017). Nonetheless, the communication between the pulp/root canal system and the periodontium complicates the management of the involved tooth.

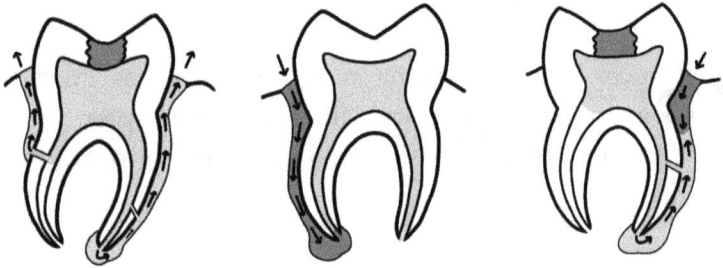

The perio-endo interface - the various routes of communication

Communication through dentin exposure can happen due to several factors, such as developmental grooves, congenital lack of cementum resulting in exposed tubules, gingival recession, or following post-periodontal mucosal repositioning (PMPR). Communication also often occurs via lateral and accessory canals. Radiographic indicators of these canals may include a distinct lateral lesion, a notch on the lateral surface, and the extrusion of filling material. The apical foramen serves as a further potential pathway for communication.

Signs and symptoms

The primary signs of an endo–perio lesion will be a deep periodontal pocket extending to the root apex and/or negative or altered response to pulp vitality/ sensibility tests (Kumar and Nisha, 2015).

Other signs/symptoms include radiographic evidence of bone loss in the apical or furcation region, spontaneous pain or pain on palpation/percussion, suppuration, tooth mobility, sinus tract/fistula, and crown and/ or gingival colour alterations. If the endo–perio lesion is associated with traumatic and/or iatrogenic factors, further signs might include root perforation, fracture/ cracking, or external root resorption. These can drastically impair the prognosis of the involved tooth.

A thorough history, probing, radiographic examination, and sensibility testing are essential for establishing a diagnosis.

Treatment planning

Evaluating the prognosis of a tooth before treatment is crucial. In cases where the pulp is the primary cause, the prognosis is usually predictable, but if significant periodontal damage has subsequently impacted the root canal, the prognosis becomes less certain.

Endo–perio lesions necessitate a thorough and collaborative approach to treatment. Typically, endodontic treatment (or re-treatment) should be performed first, followed by a reassessment of the periodontal condition two to three months later to complete the necessary treatment (Friedman and Stabholtz, 1999).

14.2 The perio–ortho interface

Orthodontics in patients with severe periodontitis can be challenging, and evidence-based guidelines should be closely followed to ensure safe and predictable results. The importance of achieving the periodontal outcomes of shallow, maintainable pockets and control of inflammation before considering orthodontic treatment is key. Orthodontic treatment should involve careful risk assessment and treatment planning, as well as the use of light and controlled force.

Orthodontics in Stage IV periodontitis

In terms of severity and complexity, Stage IV periodontitis shares characteristics with Stage III, but also involves anatomical and functional consequences due to tooth and periodontal attachment loss, such as tooth flaring, drifting, and bite collapse. These issues necessitate further interventions after active periodontal therapy has been completed.

The clinical practice guideline for managing Stage IV periodontitis offers evidence-based recommendations (Herrera et al, 2022). It emphasises the importance of interdisciplinary collaboration, including orthodontic treatment, to rehabilitate the compromised dentition of these patients.

Cases of Stage IV periodontitis can exhibit significant phenotypic differences due to varying patterns of periodontal breakdown, the number of missing teeth, inter-maxillary relationships, and the condition of the residual alveolar ridge. These factors contribute to different levels of functional and aesthetic compromise, as well as distinct treatment requirements. When discussing orthodontic management, the guidance document highlights Case Type 2, which pertains to patients experiencing pathological tooth migration characterised by elongation, drifting, and flaring, all of which can be corrected orthodontically.

Orthodontic treatment can be planned during the second step of care and, in some cases, during the third step. However, actual orthodontic interventions should only be initiated once the goals of periodontal treatment – such as achieving shallow, maintainable pockets and controlling periodontal inflammation – have been met. Starting treatment too early may jeopardise periodontal health.

Tooth movements

The advancement of periodontitis can lead to pathological tooth migration, which is evident through symptoms like drifting, flaring, and elongation of teeth. If this has occurred in individuals who have successfully undergone treatment for Stage IV periodontitis, orthodontic therapy may be required to enhance their dental aesthetics and functional occlusion. These patients typically have a healthy yet diminished periodontal structure, so the implications and requirements of orthodontic treatment may vary compared to those without any attachment loss (Martín et al, 2021).

It is crucial to first achieve periodontal objectives, for example shallow, maintainable pockets, and control of inflammation, before initiating orthodontic treatment. The guidelines (Herrera et al, 2022) indicate that orthodontic therapy does not significantly impact periodontal outcomes – such as probing pocket depth and clinical attachment levels, gingival inflammation, recession, or the risk of root resorption – provided the patient maintains optimal periodontal health throughout the process.

Orthodontic movements often involve intrusion, retraction, and proper alignment of teeth. The guidelines suggest that these movements are unlikely to negatively affect periodontal conditions, gingival inflammation, or gingival margin levels, and they do not significantly contribute to root resorption (Papageorgiou et al, 2021). Benefits may include improvements in the height of interdental papillae and a potential reduction in tooth mobility. Yet it is stressed that orthodontic treatment should not start until specific periodontal goals are met – specifically, no sites should have probing depths of 5 mm or more with BoP, and none should exceed 6 mm in probing depth (Sanz et al, 2020).

In patients with Stage IV periodontitis, tipped molars often result from tooth loss and periodontal attachment loss, frequently accompanied by bite collapse and reduced vertical dimension. In such cases, orthodontic treatment can help upright the molars and support any necessary restorative rehabilitation. The treatment guidelines (Herrera et al, 2022) examine whether these movements could adversely affect the involved teeth in terms of additional attachment and bone loss, but found insufficient evidence. Thus, while orthodontic treatment is an option, the results may be unpredictable.

As well as tilted and drifted teeth, patients with periodontitis may also have intrabony defects. According to guidelines for treating Stages I–III periodontitis, these defects should be addressed during step three of periodontal therapy through surgical regenerative procedures. When patients undergo orthodontic therapy, tooth movements may occur through the regenerated tissues. The guidelines suggest that combined orthodontic treatment can be safely administered to the affected teeth. In fact, orthodontics is shown to significantly improve periodontal outcomes and decrease gingival inflammation. There is strong evidence indicating that both short (one month) and extended (six months) intervals between periodontal regenerative treatment and orthodontic therapy yield comparable results, suggesting that a long healing period after regenerative procedures is unnecessary before starting orthodontics (Kloukos et al, 2021; Papageorgiou et al, 2021). It is important to note, though, that in terms of timing the grading is a B, indicating a recommendation rather than a strong endorsement, due to limitations in the existing studies.

Biomechanics

The application of orthodontic forces leads to immediate changes in the stress–strain distribution within the periodontal ligament (Kothiwale et al, 2020). This is accompanied by the bending of the alveolar bone, a phenomenon known as the 'cone effect'. The cone effect arises when a force is resolved into horizontal and vertical components upon application to an inclined plane. Specifically, horizontal forces induce an extrusive component that, in healthy conditions, is regulated by the supracrestal fibres (O'Leary et al, 2021). In teeth affected by periodontal disease, where bone support is compromised, the distribution of stresses and strains occurs over a reduced surface area. As a result, the resistance provided by the alveolar crest diminishes, leading to a more pronounced extrusive component. For patients with periodontitis, who may have already experienced tooth extrusion, maintaining control over vertical movement is especially vital.

In individuals with diminished periodontal support, the centre of resistance shifts further apically (Lindhe et al, 2015). This means that any force applied at the crown level causing tooth movement has a significant rotational component, making tipping movements easier to achieve. When tipping occurs, the distribution of stress and strain becomes uneven, with concentrations peaking at the coronal and apical regions. Elevated force levels pose a risk of obstructing capillary vessels, leading to hyalinisation, which is associated with indirect bone resorption and root resorption (Kothiwale et al, 2020). As such, you should apply light, controlled forces on these teeth to mitigate risks.

The bone support for periodontally affected teeth is not only reduced in the vertical dimension but also often in the buccolingual dimension (Lindhe et al, 2015). This reduction heightens the risk of hyalinisation, which can cause indirect resorption from the periodontium, ultimately diminishing vertical height and resulting in irreversible bone damage. For this reason, you must consider carefully the force levels applied for specific tooth movements.

Therefore, the biomechanical principles guiding orthodontic tooth movement in patients with periodontitis, who maintain a healthy but reduced periodontium, differ from those in healthy patients without attachment loss. To the greatest extent possible, the activation of the periodontal ligament must be limited in the teeth targeted for movement. The force applied should be minimal, and loads should be evenly distributed, focusing on root-controlled movements.

Fixed or removable?

Orthodontic tooth movements can be performed using either fixed appliances (such as braces) or removable options (like removable plates and thermoplastic aligners). In patients with advanced periodontitis who require orthodontic treatment to improve or maintain periodontal stability, fixed appliances are generally recommended over removable ones (Watanabe et al, 2020).

Removable clear aligners are popular due to their aesthetic appeal and ease of maintaining oral hygiene compared to fixed appliances (Miller et al, 2021). But traditional braces have long been accepted by adults, and there are now more aesthetically pleasing options available for fixed appliances, including ceramic brackets and lingual braces.

For patients with Stage IV periodontitis who have a healthy but reduced periodontium, anchorage can often pose challenges. In these cases, you could consider skeletal anchorage devices, such as implants or temporary anchorage devices (TADs) like mini-screws or mini-plates, as potentially valuable adjuncts to enhance the effectiveness of orthodontic therapy and improve periodontal outcomes (Diem et al, 2019). While some patients may experience discomfort with temporary anchorage devices, this has not been thoroughly investigated in the literature.

Management of complications

Orthodontic appliances can lead to increased microbial colonisation and biofilm retention, making it essential to implement a comprehensive oral hygiene and supportive periodontal management protocol throughout the course of orthodontic treatment. This approach is crucial for maintaining periodontal health and preventing adverse effects, such as enamel demineralisation, tooth discolouration, and additional loss of periodontal support, including the formation of periodontal abscesses and subsequent bone loss (Keller et al, 2021). Professional biofilm control and other SPC should be tailored to the patient's risk profile and clearly communicated during the consent process (Kumar et al, 2020a).

During orthodontic therapy, you must closely monitor the patient's periodontal condition at each appointment. If there are any signs of periodontal relapse or recurrence, active orthodontic treatment must be paused. The affected teeth should be maintained passively while the necessary periodontal treatment is provided and you reinforce a good oral regime. Once periodontal health and stability have been restored, active orthodontic therapy can resume (Hassan et al, 2019).

Gingival enlargement is more commonly associated with fixed orthodontic appliances but can also occur with aligner systems. This enlargement may impede the completion of orthodontic treatment. If it occurs, it is vital that you communicate the importance of optimal oral hygiene; you can perform a gingivectomy if necessary. Typically, if key periodontal parameters remain stable, the procedure would be carried out after the completion of orthodontic treatment (García et al, 2020).

As previously noted, orthodontic treatment doesn't inherently increase the risk of root resorption in patients with periodontitis. Apical root resorption is thought to result from a combination of individual biological variability and mechanical factors. This complication is more common with fixed appliances compared to removable ones and tends to occur in cases with longer treatment durations (Keller et al, 2021). Although periodontal factors don't seem to influence the likelihood of root resorption, its impact in periodontitis patients with significant bone loss is an important consideration from an anchorage perspective. If root resorption is detected and progresses significantly, orthodontic treatment may need to be halted if the risks outweigh the benefits. Generally, no specific treatment is required unless the affected tooth or teeth lose vitality. If increased mobility is observed, permanent retention through a fixed retainer may be necessary (Hassan et al, 2019).

Maintenance and retention

Relapse after orthodontic treatment towards pre-treatment positions is common, particularly in patients with compromised periodontal health. This relapse can lead to both aesthetic and functional issues, undermining treatment outcomes and patient satisfaction (Bishara et al, 2018). For this reason, life-long SPC and orthodontic retention are crucial after the completion of orthodontic treatment. These pro-tocols should be tailored based on the individual patient's needs and risk factors (Kumar et al, 2020a).

In summary, evidence supports the use of appro-priately designed, permanent fixed passive retain-ers, which may be used alone or in conjunction with removable retainers. Even so, fixed retainers can be susceptible to issues like retention failure, increased plaque accumulation, and unintentional tooth move-ments due to distortion of the bonded wire (Mason et al, 2019). As a result, lifelong supportive measures are crucial to detect early retainer failures, such as par-tial debonds, to monitor any undesired tooth move-ments, and to assess periodontal stability (Kumar et al, 2020b). Additionally, consider the option of remov-able clear retainers worn at night, for better retention and patient comfort.

15
Pocket Reduction Surgery

In the 1970s and 1980s, research established that non-surgical periodontal therapy is effective at reducing inflammation in deep periodontal pockets and improves clinical attachment levels (Caffesse et al, 1986). But even with diligent efforts, residual biofilm and calculus often remain. As such, surgical intervention might be necessary in cases where inflammation persists even after non-surgical treatment (Haffajee and Socransky, 1994).

Historically, periodontal surgery aimed to remove diseased tissue, primarily by excising diseased gingival tissue and what was thought to be necrotic bone (Cobb, 1996). Understanding evolved with the recognition that periodontal disease does not cause bone necrosis; rather, gingival inflammation and bone loss are a defensive response to bacterial infection (Nyman et al, 1982). As a result, the focus shifted towards pocket elimination as the primary goal of periodontal therapy, leading to the adoption of procedures such as gingivectomy and apically positioned flap techniques to eliminate pockets and allow access for scaling and improved oral hygiene (Löe, 1988).

By the 1980s, advancements in our understanding of periodontal biology, disease pathogenesis, and wound-healing mechanisms led to a re-evaluation of the need for pocket elimination. The focus shifted again, this time towards obtaining access to the root surfaces for effective debridement and creating gingival contours that facilitate effective self-performed biofilm control (Karnik et al, 1999).

Access flaps, which include various techniques developed over nearly a century – such as the original Widman flap (1918), the Neumann flap (1920), the modified flap operation by Kirkland (1931), the apically repositioned flap described by Friedman (1962), and the modified Widman flap introduced by Ramfjord and Nissle (1974) – enabled thorough access to root surfaces, root concavities, and furcations. The choice of surgical technique in the 1970s and 1980s often reflected the philosophy of different dental schools. Numerous clinical trials during this period showed that in patients with excellent oral hygiene, the specific surgical technique employed to access root surfaces had minimal impact on long-term outcomes (Socransky et al, 1984).

By contrast, patients with poor plaque control continued to experience attachment loss, regardless of the surgical method used (Cobb, 1996).

It became evident that successful post-operative plaque control is essential for maintaining the periodontal environment after surgery. In addition, patient-related factors, including compliance and smoking, were identified as crucial influences on periodontal wound healing and overall treatment outcomes (Tornes et al, 2005).

In recent years, advancements in periodontal surgical techniques have been helped by the development of innovative instruments and the application of illumination and magnification. Minimally invasive surgical approaches and microsurgical techniques are currently under investigation, potentially offering benefits in terms of wound healing, reduced recession, and decreased patient morbidity (Sgolastra et al, 2016).

15.1 Key aims and considerations

The three main aims of pocket reduction surgery are to:

1. Allow access and visibility for adequate debridement

2. Establish a favourable dentogingival architecture to support oral hygiene

3. Reduce probing depths and possibly restore periodontal apparatus when there has been attachment loss

Before proceeding with any surgical intervention, it is essential to have completed at least one but ideally two sessions of non-surgical periodontal therapy (subgingival PMPR). This initial treatment phase allows for the elimination of local risk factors and provides an opportunity to evaluate the patient's oral hygiene practices and compliance. After non-surgical therapy, the periodontal tissues typically exhibit reduced inflammation, which allows better management of the surgical flap. Many periodontal cases can be effectively managed non-surgically, and so this approach should always be the first line of treatment (Garg, Ranjan, and Ranjan, 2022).

Engaging the patient in their care is crucial, as optimal biofilm control is necessary to prevent deterioration of the periodontal condition post-surgery (Nyman et al, 1977). As discussed earlier, healing outcomes can be particularly poor in smokers; therefore, surgical interventions are often postponed in these patients (Scabbia et al, 2001). It is also vital to consider any systemic conditions or bleeding disorders that may affect surgical outcomes. Adequate bone support is required for successful surgery, and the pattern of bone loss will influence the choice of surgical technique, with procedures typically focused on localised sites (Garg et al, 2022; Aapeng et al, 2023).

The concept of critical probing depth can guide clinical decision-making in periodontal therapy (Lindhe et al, 1982). This principle suggests a threshold probing depth, above which surgical intervention may lead to attachment gain, and below which the risk of attachment loss increases. Flap surgery is generally indicated when probing depths exceed 5.4 mm, while non-surgical options are preferred for depths ranging from 2.9 to 5.4 mm (Wagner and Gmür, 1993; McGuire and Nunn, 1996). Clinicians often round this number, commonly considering surgery for probing depths of 6 mm or more (Müller and Heine, 2019).

All surgical procedures typically result in a reduction of probing depths, with the extent of this reduction being positively correlated with the initial pocket depth. Although short-term results following surgery show greater depth reduction compared to non-surgical treatment, long-term outcomes (five to eight years) can vary significantly (Cortellini et al, 2017).

15.2 Surgical details

Persistence of large probing depths following active periodontal therapy is associated with an increased probability of tooth loss, so surgery may be used to address this. Pocket reduction surgery may be resective or regenerative.

The overall steps in either type of pocket reduction surgery can be summarised as follows:

1. Flap design/incisions

2. Removal of excised tissues (if resective surgery)

3. Raise flap

4. Debride root surfaces and bony defects

5. Management of bone

6. Check flap apposition and adjust if needed

7. Suturing

Probing after non-surgical treatment can be performed after two months. For pocket reduction surgery, it's important to wait three months for a resective case and six months for a regenerative case. A radiograph should also be taken for a regenerative case to assess evidence of bony infill.

Various resective surgical techniques exist, and are primarily employed when there is horizontal bone loss. Once a flap is elevated, procedures such as osteoplasty or ostectomy may be performed to enhance the bony architecture, facilitating better tissue adaptation during suturing. In the anterior regions, a papilla preservation flap (Cortellini and Tonetti, 2005) is often used to maintain the interdental soft tissue and maximise coverage. Typically, healing occurs through the formation of a long junctional epithelium.

Regenerative therapies have been increasingly applied to enhance clinical outcomes, particularly in areas with intrabony defects, which are associated with a higher risk of disease progression. The guidelines from the EFP (Sanz et al, 2020) recommend periodontal regenerative surgery for teeth showing residual deep pockets of 3 mm or more, particularly where this is in conjunction with intrabony defects. The benefits of a regenerative approach include improved aesthetics, a more conservative treatment strategy, enhanced clinical outcomes, long-term stability, and fewer complications compared to traditional resective surgeries. However, regenerative procedures may not be appropriate for every case and can be sensitive to technique.

Periodontal breakdown results in three types of defects: suprabony (horizontal), intrabony (vertical), and interradicular (furcation) defects. Regenerative surgery is indicated for intrabony and interradicular defects, when deemed suitable. Optimal outcomes are generally observed in deep, narrow defects with three walls (Trombelli et al, 2013). Significant mobility can hinder healing, necessitating splinting if mobility is considerable (Aroca and Mombelli, 2015). Additionally, any compromised endodontic status should be addressed before proceeding with surgery, as it may affect outcomes (Vignoletti and Sanz, 2014). For furcation involvement, clinical improvements can be anticipated in mandibular Grade 2 defects (Greenstein and Cavallaro, 2006).

Successful regeneration relies on the coordinated development of new alveolar bone, dental cementum, and a functionally oriented periodontal ligament that interposes these two tissues. Key facilitators of this process are site protection, maintenance of space, and stability of the blood clot (Trombelli et al, 2014).

BONE GRAFTING DEFINITIONS

- **Osteogenic:** New bone formation occurs as a result of bone-forming cells contained in graft, eg enamel matrix derivative, autogenous bone

- **Osteoinductive:** Bone formation induced in surrounding soft tissue immediately adjacent to grafted material, eg demineralised freeze-dried bone allograft (DFDBA)

- **Osteoconductive:** Graft material does not directly contribute to new bone formation but serves as a scaffold for bone formation by adjacent host bone, eg freeze-dried bone allograft (FDBA), B-TCP

- **Autografts:** Tissues transferred from one part of the body to another part of the same person

- **Allogenic:** Harvested from genetically distinct individuals within the same species, eg freeze-dried undermineralised/demineralised bone allograft

- **Xenogenic:** Harvested from species genetically different from humans, eg bovine anorganic cancellous bone, Bio-Oss®

- **Alloplastic:** Biologic materials that are synthesised or chemically processed, eg beta tricalcium phosphate, porous hydroxyapatite, non-porous

hydroxyapatite, HTR polymer, bio-active glasses and ceramics
- **Guided tissue regeneration (GTR):** Attempt to control cells repopulating site by placing a barrier membrane during wound healing to prevent epithelial and connective tissue growth

Several materials have been proposed for use with regenerative therapy. Below are key facts about the main ones used in practice.

Enamel matrix derivative

- Product: Emdogain, Straumann.

- Gel formation.

- Enamel matrix proteins produced by Hertwig's root sheath have been shown to support regenerative processes. This purified fraction is obtained from the enamel layer of developing porcine teeth (Stern et al, 2009).

- The primary component of these proteins is amelogenin. This is a hydrophobic protein that comprises over 90% of the total protein content, along with other proteins such as enamelin and ameloblastin. Amelogenin acts as a cell-adhesion matrix-bound protein and is believed to function as an epithelial-mesenchymal signalling molecule, effectively mimicking the biological events that take place during root development and promoting periodontal regeneration (Bartlett et al, 2013).

- These proteins play a crucial role in wound healing, enhancing soft tissue regeneration, and supporting angiogenic activity (Bichara et al, 2017).

- Enamel matrix derivatives significantly affect the behaviour of various cell types by facilitating processes such as cell attachment, spreading, proliferation, differentiation, and survival. They also influence the expression of key transcription factors, growth factors, cytokines, and other important molecules (Nanci et al, 2019).

Bio-Oss®

- Product produced by Geistlich.

- Bovine-derived natural bone substitute.

- The osteoconductive characteristics of Bio-Oss contribute to effective and reliable bone regeneration. The particles of Bio-Oss integrate seamlessly into the newly formed bone matrix, helping to maintain volume over an extended period (Schlegel et al, 2015).

- Subsequent application of a Bio-Gide® collagen membrane enables undisturbed regeneration in the augmented area (Hämmerle and Trombelli, 2017).

Bio-Gide®

- Product produced by Geistlich.
- Porcine-derived collagen membrane that is resorbable.
- Due to its bilayer structure, the membrane not only prevents the ingrowth of soft tissue into the augmented site but also acts as a guide for the appropriate cascade of bone, soft tissue and blood vessel development (Buser et al, 2015).

Among the various materials employed today, there is currently evidence of true periodontal regeneration (periodontal ligament, cementum, and bone) for decalcified freeze-dried bone allograft, demineralised bovine bone mineral (Bio-Oss), and enamel matrix derivative (Emdogain) (Sanz et al, 2020). By contrast, bioactive glass, hydroxyapatite, and tricalcium phosphate, although efficient for improving clinical parameters, have histologically shown limited evidence of regeneration. The regenerative effect has been demonstrated for platelet-derived factors, but there is currently no histologic evidence for periodontal regeneration for autogenous platelet-rich plasma and platelet-rich fibrin.

According to the systematic review by Nibali et al (2019), enamel matrix derivative in combination with papillary preservation flaps is the treatment of choice for residual pockets with deep (≥3 mm) intra-bony defects. For wider defects, consider the addition of demineralised bone matrix.

The surgical techniques used in regenerative therapy have evolved towards more microsurgical and minimally invasive approaches. These less traumatic methods enable careful flap preparation and suturing, resulting in reduced tissue damage. Consequently, this facilitates quicker and more effective integration of new capillary buds from the recipient site with the severed vessels of the graft or flap. Employing papillary preservation flaps has also been shown to improve clinical outcomes and should be seen as a crucial prerequisite for any regenerative procedure (Huang et al, 2017; Yamada et al, 2020).

16

Gingival Recession And Surgery

As well as pocket reduction, there are surgical treatment options for gingival recession.

Gingival recession refers to the apical displacement of the gingival margin, which results in the exposure of the tooth root. This condition can adversely affect aesthetic outcomes and is among the primary reasons patients seek periodontal treatment. The severity and extent of recession can vary significantly, and its impact on individuals is case-specific. The development of gingival recession is not an inevitable consequence of age, but it is, to a degree, a reflection of some pathological change (Khan et al, 2016).

16.1 Aetiology

The aetiology of gingival recession is multifaceted, often involving both predisposing and precipitating factors. Predisposing factors heighten a patient's risk, while precipitating factors act as triggers for the onset of recession.

A critical predisposing factor related to soft tissue is the presence of a thin phenotype. When the probe can be seen shining through the gingival tissue during probing, this indicates a thin phenotype. Individuals with a thin phenotype typically have more delicate gingiva compared to those with a thick phenotype, making them more susceptible to recession (Baker et al, 2018). Other soft-tissue factors include high frenal attachments and shallow vestibular depths. Hard tissue factors contributing to recession include thin buccal bone, as well as the presence of dehiscences or fenestrations. The positioning of teeth within the arch, whether anatomical or because of orthodontic treatment, along with a mismatch between root size and bone width, can also influence the likelihood of developing gingival recession. Finally, a loss of interproximal bone support is a significant contributor to this condition (Trombelli, 2015).

The two main precipitating factors associated with gingival recession are trauma and plaque accumulation. One of the most common forms of trauma is aggressive brushing, typically resulting in buccal recession without loss of interdental soft tissue. Other forms of trauma include flossing techniques that may lead to Stillman's clefts, as well as habits like nail biting or picking at the gum line. Tongue and lip piercings can contribute to recession in their respective areas. Trauma can also arise from malocclusion, such as an overbite that causes injury to the palate or severe Class II Division 2 malocclusions. Inadequate biofilm control may lead to inflammation, further exacerbating gingival recession.

As clinicians, it is our responsibility to identify these contributing factors and manage the modifiable ones, regardless of whether surgical interventions are necessary. For instance, if aggressive brushing is not recognised and corrected, any periodontal plastic surgery performed will likely not yield long-term success (Zhang et al, 2021).

16.2 Classification

Previously, gingival recession was classified using Miller's classification (Miller, 1985). The latest classification system (Jepsen et al, 2018) divides gingival recession into three different recession types (RT), as follows:

- **RT1:** Gingival recession with no loss of interproximal attachment. Interproximal CEJ is clinically not detectable in either mesial or distal aspects of the tooth.

- **RT2:** Gingival recession associated with loss of interproximal attachment. The amount of interproximal attachment loss is less than or equal to the buccal attachment.

- **RT3:** Gingival recession associated with loss of interproximal attachment. The amount of interproximal attachment loss is higher than the buccal attachment loss.

Further detail can be added on the depth of the recession, gingival thickness, keratinised tissue width, presence of a detectable CEJ, and the existence of a root surface concavity.

16.3 Pathogenesis

The mechanism behind trauma-induced gingival recession is fundamentally different from that in gingival recession caused by bacterial factors. In cases of trauma-induced recession, the causative agent affects the external gingival surface, initially leading to gingival abrasion. With ongoing trauma, the combined effect of direct tissue damage and secondary inflammatory responses damages the gingival connective tissue, resulting in the formation of a gingival ulcer. If the damage extends through the full thickness of the gingival connective tissue, the root dehiscence becomes exposed. This process, called centripetal, progresses from the exterior towards the interior.

16.4 Treatment

In all instances, it is essential to address the modifiable aetiological factors. For example, if excessive brushing is a primary contributing factor, schedule an appointment specifically aimed at teaching gentle yet effective home care practices. When surgical intervention is not clearly indicated, or the patient is hesitant, careful monitoring of the gingival recession becomes critical. This can be accomplished through regular six-point recession measurements, along with photographic documentation and scanning, typically every six to twelve months. Should there be signs of progression, surgical intervention might then become necessary.

Surgery may be indicated for aesthetic purposes, to augment keratinised tissue/tissue thickness and prevent progression of the gingival recession. Decision-making should be based on: patient factors, aesthetic requirements, need for gingival augmentation, single/multiple defects, defect anatomy, and need for orthodontics. The following factors will negatively affect the predictability of root coverage: reduction in level of interdental support, short papillae height, tooth rotation, tooth extrusion, large defects, convex root surfaces, flap tension and poor patient compliance.

Several surgical techniques exist. Pedicle soft-tissue graft procedures include:

- Rotational flap procedures
    - Laterally sliding flap
    - Double papilla flap
    - Oblique rotational flap

- Advanced flap procedures
    - Coronally advanced flap
    - Semilunar coronally repositioned flap

- Regenerative procedures
- Tunnelling

Free soft-tissue graft procedures include:

- Epithelised graft
- Subepithelial connective tissue graft

Free gingival graft

The free gingival graft is often employed to enhance the height of keratinised tissue, thicken gingival tissue, and deepen the vestibule. Although root coverage is not consistently achievable, the main aim of this procedure is to promote periodontal health rather than improve aesthetics. This results in a more resilient gum tissue ('tough gum') that protects the tooth and makes cleaning more comfortable, thereby minimising the risk of further recession. The graft material is harvested from the patient's palate.

Coronally advanced flap

The coronally advanced flap is a pedicle soft-tissue graft procedure based on a coronal shift of the soft tissues on the exposed root surface. It is the treatment of choice for isolated recession defects. The most recent version of this technique uses a trapezoidal flap design and a split–full–split-thickness flap elevation approach (Cortellini and Bissada, 2018). The split or partial thickness elevation at the level of the surgical papilla provides anchorage and blood supply to the interproximal areas, as well as improving blending in terms of colour and thickness (Cairo et al, 2018). The full-thickness elevation of the soft tissue apical to the root exposure confers the maximum flap thickness and, thus, creates a better opportunity to achieve root coverage to the portion of the flap residing over the exposed avascular root surface. The more apical split-thickness flap elevation facilitates the coronal displacement of the flap (Tonetti and Jepsen, 2014).

There is extensive evidence supporting the use of root coverage procedures in the treatment of localised gingival recession defects, but few studies reporting the outcomes for the treatment of multiple gingival recessions. The coronally advanced flap for multiple recession defects was introduced by Zucchelli and De Sanctis (2000) as a novel approach to treat more than two adjacent teeth with gingival recession. This technique comprises an envelope type of flap (with no vertical releasing incisions) that anticipates the rotational movement of the surgical papillae during the coronal advancement of the flap (Cortellini and Bissada, 2018). When there are multiple recession defects in one area, it is best to treat them all with one procedure rather than focusing on the deepest defect alone. Coronally advanced flaps are often used in conjunction with a connective tissue graft sandwiched underneath. This is common when there is a lack of keratinised tissue, or the flap is thin (Baldi et al, 1999). Covering the graft increases the blood supply, and the aesthetic outcome is improved by hiding the white-scar appearance of the grafted tissue.

Alternative materials to the palatal connective tissue graft are available but these are likely to be less predictable (Tinti et al, 1992). Treatment of multiple recession defects with coronally advanced flaps with or without connective tissue grafts can have a considerable impact on periodontal and overall smile aesthetics. Often, a combined restorative approach is required in cases of abrasive tooth wear.

Other

In the '90s, the tunnel procedure for root coverage was introduced (Allen, 1994). The unique feature of this procedure is that the interdental papillae are left intact. A connective tissue graft is placed in the tunnel, and it does not need to be completely covered if the dimension of the graft is sufficient to ensure graft survival. The main proposed benefit of the technique is the minimally invasive nature of the surgery. Recently, the tunnel technique was modified to include coronal positioning of the marginal tissue, which allows complete coverage of the graft.

Currently, there is a lack of good-quality evidence for other procedures, such as the 'pinhole' surgical technique.

Healing

Tissue graft procedures are best suited to those with good bone levels and interdental support. Healing for these types of surgery involves a mix of repair and regeneration. Shallow probing depths occur. The surgical results are likely to last sufficiently (enough to not have to repeat the surgery), provided the aetiological factors have been addressed (Tonetti and Jepsen, 2014).

17
Crown-Lengthening Surgery

Another type of surgical treatment under the periodontal umbrella is crown lengthening, commonly referred to by patients as a 'gum lift'. This aims to resolve gingival excess and might be offered for either aesthetic or functional reasons.

17.1 Definition and indications

Crown lengthening has been described by Cohen et al (2007) as the surgical removal of hard and soft periodontal tissue to gain supragingival tooth length, allowing for longer clinical crowns and the re-establishment of the biologic width. The term biologic width is no longer used, replaced by 'supracrestal tissue attachment' in the updated periodontal classification (Jepsen et al, 2018). This encompasses the junctional epithelium and supracrestal connective tissue. According to Garguilo, Wentz, and Orban (1961), this should be approximately 2 mm. If the supracrestal tissue attachment is not respected or recreated, this will result in the unwanted consequences of gingival inflammation, pocketing recession, and/or bone loss.

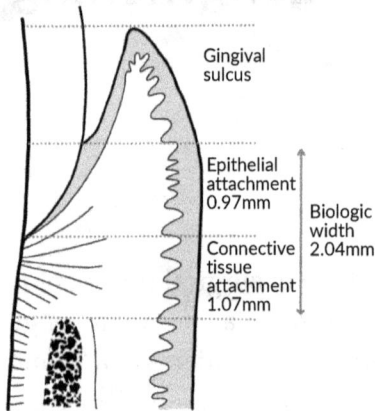

The supracrestal tissue attachment is made up of the junctional epithelium and supracrestal connective tissue

Crown-lengthening procedures are divided into two main categories: aesthetic and restorative/functional. Aesthetic crown lengthening aims to address issues such as excessive gingival display, short clinical crowns, and uneven gingival contours. On the other hand, restorative or functional crown lengthening is necessary when there is insufficient sound tooth structure available for restoration, to gain access to subgingival fractures, caries, or perforations, or to reposition crown margins that infringe upon the supracrestal tissue attachment.

17.2 Ideal 'pink' aesthetics

A smile is generally described as 'pleasant' when it exposes all of the maxillary teeth along with approximately 1 mm of facial gingiva. Gingival exposure of up to 2–3 mm is normally found acceptable, whereas patients are usually dissatisfied with any greater exposure (> 3 mm) (Garber and Salama, 1996). Patients with a high smile line who expose a large band of gingiva may be classified as having a 'gummy' smile.

The ideal gingival architecture consists of several features:

- **Gingival zenith position:** The gingival zenith refers to the lowest point of the gingival contour. According to Chu et al (2009), the gingival zeniths for maxillary central incisors should ideally be positioned about 1 mm distal to the crown's midline. For lateral incisors, the zenith should be approximately 0.4 mm distal, while the zenith for canines is typically aligned centrally along the long axis.

- **Relative gingival margins:** In terms of apico-coronal positioning, the zeniths of the lateral incisors should be positioned 1 mm coronal to those of the central incisors and canines.

- **The gingival aesthetic line:** This is the line connecting the tangents of the zeniths of the central incisors and canines. The angle formed at the intersection of this line with the maxillary dental midline is referred to as the gingival aesthetic line angle, with the ideal angle ranging between 45 to 90 degrees. Achieving gingival symmetry between the right and left sides of the mouth is also a key aesthetic consideration.

Lastly, it is important to take into account the ideal height-to-width ratios for teeth: the central incisor should be at 80%, the lateral incisor at 70%, and the canine at 75% (Gargiulo et al, 2006).

17.3 Causes of gingival excess

Before considering crown lengthening, a proper diagnosis is essential. The latest classification scheme categorises gingival excess under mucogingival deformities and conditions, encompassing various anatomical factors (Cairo et al, 2018). Several causes can contribute to this condition, either individually or in combination. The most prevalent factors include altered passive eruption, dentoalveolar extrusion due to tooth wear, vertical maxillary excess, and a short or hypermobile upper lip (Cortellini and Bissada, 2018).

Identifying the specific cause(s) is crucial since not all cases are appropriate for aesthetic crown-lengthening procedures. For instance, vertical maxillary excess may necessitate maxillofacial surgery for resolution, while a hypermobile lip could benefit from interventions such as botulinum toxin injections or lip-repositioning surgery (Cairo et al, 2018).

Altered passive eruption is one of the conditions most frequently addressed through aesthetic crown lengthening. This condition is relatively common, affecting approximately 35% of the population (Cairo et al, 2018). The process begins after the complete eruption of the tooth's anatomical crown and is characterised by the apical migration of the dentogingival junction. As the epithelial attachment moves apically, the length of the clinical crown increases until the junction reaches a physiological distance of 0.5–2.0 mm coronal to the cementoenamel junction (CEJ). If the dentogingival junction does not retract adequately during this passive phase, it results in altered or delayed passive eruption (Goldman and Cohen, 1971).

Coslet, Vanarsdall, and Weisgold (1977) proposed a classification system based on the relationship between the gingiva and the underlying alveolar bone. Evaluating the position of the gingival margin in relation to the CEJ and buccal bone crest, along with the relationships between the crown, root, and alveolar crest, is essential to determine whether the observed gingival excess, or 'gummy' smile, is due to altered passive eruption.

17.4 Treatment sequence

With crown lengthening, the planning phase is the most important. Understanding key factors, such as where the reference point is and the amount of bone removal required, is critical. The surgery itself may include both soft and hard tissue adjustment. It's also imperative that you understand the restorative phase in terms of when and where you can provisionalise and definitively restore, if required.

The treatment sequence for crown lengthening typically consists of three stages:

1. Planning

2. The surgery itself

3. Further restorative treatment

Planning

The planning stage for aesthetic crown lengthening plays a vital role in achieving a successful long-term outcome and aligning with patient expectations. Initially, it is essential to establish or maintain periodontal health and effective plaque control prior to the procedure. If a patient has been diagnosed with gingivitis or periodontitis through a comprehensive periodontal assessment, these conditions must be addressed before proceeding. Additionally, local factors such as the crown-to-root ratio, furcation entrance level, root proximity, and the tooth's endodontic condition should be evaluated and any necessary endodontic treatment should be completed prior to crown lengthening.

Next, it is crucial to identify the reference point or finish line for the procedure. In cases of altered passive eruption, the CEJ is typically used as the reference point, but it can also be based on existing or provisional restorations or guided by a surgical stent. For aesthetic cases, understanding the principles of 'pink' aesthetics and assessing the current gingival architecture will help you to determine the extent of crown lengthening required for the relevant teeth. Considering facial symmetry, such as the interpupillary line, can provide you with further insight.

The extent of crown lengthening may also depend on the restorative treatment plan. Discussing with the patient their aesthetic expectations will allow you to ensure that these are realistic before surgery. Visual aids like annotated photographs, in-mouth composite mock-ups, and wax-ups can assist in this process, along with digital smile design. Cone-beam computed tomography (CBCT) scans can also be beneficial for diagnostic purposes, although currently they are not commonly used solely for crown-lengthening treatment planning.

Assessing the amount of keratinised tissue is critical, as it will inform the surgical approach, whether resective, apically positioned, or a combination of both. Ideally, at least 2 mm of keratinised tissue should remain after surgery – which is more comfortable compared to having only lining mucosa – to help the patient maintain optimal plaque control.

The position of the bone and the distance from the bone level to the reference point will dictate whether any bone removal is necessary. The supracrestal tissue attachment should ideally be about 2 mm, so when considering the depth of the gingival sulcus, there should be approximately 3 mm between the reference point and the bone level. If this measurement is already met, bone removal is not required; otherwise, it must be performed to prevent invasion of the supracrestal tissue attachment and its related negative effects. High-quality periapical radiographs and bone-sounding techniques will aid you in assessing the bone position. You can also use gutta-percha points alongside radiographs to obtain valuable information regarding the clinical and anatomical crown height relative to the bone level. In many cases, raising a flap will help to definitively determine the bone level and its architecture.

The surgery

The procedure used for aesthetic crown lengthening typically involves elevating only a buccal flap and necessitates the exclusive removal of buccal bone. By contrast, restorative or functional crown lengthening requires the elevation of both buccal and palatal/lingual flaps, as bone removal is generally required on all surfaces. Initially, bleeding points are managed, followed by a superficial scoring incision in the epithelium. Once you are satisfied with the initial incision, make a full-thickness incision. To minimise the risk of developing 'black triangles', the interproximal tissue can be thinned instead of fully reflected or preserved by excluding it from the flap design. Vertical incisions are typically avoided to reduce the potential for scarring. You can use a 15c blade or a laser for the incisions, depending on preference.

If bone removal, particularly ostectomy, is necessary, the objective is to eliminate sufficient bone to re-establish the supracrestal tissue attachment. Additionally, it is essential to create a gradual contour of the osseous crest to restore positive architecture, which may also require osteoplasty. Any visible bony exostoses that become apparent during smiling should also be addressed through osteoplasty. Bone removal can be carried out using a suitable anti-retraction micromotor or piezoelectric handpieces/burs, potentially supplemented with hand chisels or curettes.

The suturing technique typically employed is either single interrupted or mattress sutures. In aesthetic cases where eversion of the gingival tissue is necessary (to prevent black triangles), an internal mattress suture is ideal. If the papilla is wide or a diastema is present, a horizontal internal mattress suture is preferred; for narrow papillae, a vertical internal mattress suture is more appropriate. Fine sutures, such as 5–0 or 6–0, promote optimal healing. The choice of suture material ultimately depends on your preference.

Unlike restorative or functional crown lengthening, periodontal dressings are not utilised in aesthetic crown-lengthening cases. Sutures are typically removed about two weeks after the surgical procedure. Advise the patient to take regular analgesics as needed, maintain a soft diet for four to five days, and use an antiseptic mouth rinse while avoiding brushing the surgical site for two weeks. In cases of altered passive eruption, only the crown of the tooth is usually exposed, while in other situations, particularly restorative cases, some root exposure may occur. Sensitivity is generally not a concern, so no additional measures are typically necessary during the two-week recovery period.

Further restorative treatment

In cases of altered passive eruption, restorative work after surgery is not always necessary unless the patient has a specific desire to enhance the aesthetics of the tooth. When crown lengthening has been performed for other restorative purposes, such as addressing tooth wear due to dentoalveolar extrusion, a subsequent restorative phase is generally anticipated. Provisional restorations can be placed after the removal of sutures; however, for teeth located in the aesthetic zone, it may be prudent to delay definitive restorations for around six months, as the position of the gingival crest may continue to evolve during this time. Consequently, lab-fabricated provisional restorations are frequently utilised during this interim period. For other restorative cases, waiting about three months before proceeding with definitive restorations may be advisable.

Coronal displacement of the gingival margin tends to be more significant in individuals with thick gingival phenotypes, but it is essential to obtain informed consent from the patient regarding the possibility of revision surgery. Typically, if revision is needed and the bone level is appropriately positioned, a gingivectomy may suffice.

Conclusion

As we reach the conclusion of this comprehensive guide to modern periodontics, I hope you feel armed with a robust foundation in the essential concepts and practices that define this vital field. Throughout this book, I have aimed to provide a clear, concise, and practical resource that enhances your ability to deliver exceptional periodontal care.

By delving into the foundations of periodontal disease, mastering the art of assessment and diagnosis, and exploring a wide range of treatment strategies, you should now be well-equipped to address the myriad challenges that may arise in your professional practice. The advanced topics covered in the final sections ensure that you are well-versed in the latest developments and techniques and can confidently handle even the most complex cases.

My goal has been to empower you with knowledge and tools that will translate directly into improved patient outcomes. Whether you are integrating new techniques into your routine, managing a periodontal emergency, or planning a surgical intervention, this guide is designed to support you every step of the way.

Thank you for choosing this book as your trusted companion in your professional journey. It will serve as a valuable reference, continually aiding you in providing the highest standard of care to your patients. As you apply these insights and techniques, may you find both professional fulfilment and success in your ongoing commitment to excellence in periodontics.

References

The Periodontium And Beyond

Chapple, ILC, 'Time to take periodontitis seriously', *British Medical Journal*, 348 (2014), 2645

Chapple, ILC and Genco, R, 'Diabetes and periodontal diseases: consensus report of the Joint EFP/ AAP Workshop on Periodontitis and Systemic Diseases', *Journal of Clinical Periodontology*, 40/Suppl 14 (2013), S106–S112

GBD 2017 Disease and Injury Incidence and Prevalence Collaborators, 'Global, regional, and national incidence, prevalence, and years lived with disability for 354 diseases and injuries for 195 countries and territories, 1990–2017: A systematic analysis for the Global Burden of Disease Study 2017', *Lancet*, 392, 10159 (2018), 1789–1858

Grossi, SG et al, 'Assessment of risk for periodontal disease. I. Risk indicators for attachment loss', *Journal of Periodontology*, 65 (1994), 260–267

Hirschfeld, J and Chapple, ILC, *Periodontitis and Systemic Diseases* (Quintessence Publishing, 2021)

Jakubovics, NS et al, 'The dental plaque biofilm matrix', *Periodontology 2000*, 86/1 (2021), 32–56

Kassebaum, NJ et al, 'Global burden of severe periodontitis in 1990–2010: A systematic review and meta-regression', *Journal of Dental Research*, 93 (2014), 1045–1053

Lang, N and Lindhe, J, *Clinical Periodontology and Implant Dentistry*, 6th edition (Wiley Blackwell, 2015)

Preshaw, PM and Bissett, SM, 'Periodontitis and diabetes', *British Dental Journal*, 227 (2019), 577–584

Simpson, TC et al, 'Treatment of periodontal disease for glycaemic control in people with diabetes', *Cochrane Database of Systematic Reviews*, 12/5 (2010), CD004714

Van Dyke, TE et al, 'The nexus between periodontal inflammation and dysbiosis', *Frontiers in Immunology*, Mar 31/11 (2020), 511

Think Like A Detective

Ah, MK, Johnson, GK, Kaldahl, WB, Patil, KD, and Kalkwarf, KL, 'The effect of smoking on the response to periodontal therapy', *Journal of Clinical Periodontology*, 21 (1994), 91–97

Action on Smoking and Health (ASH), 'Use of e-cigarettes (vapes) among adults in Great Britain' (ASH, 2023), https://ash.org.uk/uploads/Use-of-e-cigarettes-among-adults-in-Great-Britain-2023.pdf, accessed 19 July 2024

Bergstrom, J and Bostrom, L, 'Tobacco smoking and periodontal hemorrhagic responsiveness', *Journal of Clinical Periodontology*, 28 (2001), 680–685

Bostrom, L, Linder, LE, and Bergstrom, J, 'Influence of smoking on the outcome of periodontal surgery: A 5-year follow-up', *Journal of Clinical Periodontology*, 25 (1998), 194–201

Chapple, ILC and Genco, R, 'Diabetes and periodontal diseases: consensus report of the Joint EFP/ AAP Workshop on Periodontitis and Systemic Diseases', *Journal of Clinical Periodontology*, 40/Suppl 14 (2013), S106–S112

European Federation of Periodontology, 'Oral health and pregnancy – key messages for oral-health professionals' (EFP), www.efp.org/fileadmin/uploads/efp/Documents/Campaigns/Oral_Health_and_Pregnancy/Brochures/key-messages-dental.pdf, accessed 19 July 2024

Holliday, R et al, 'Electronic cigarettes and oral health', *Journal of Dental Research*, 100/9 (2021), 906–913

Hugoson, A, Ljungquist, B, and Breivik, T, 'The relationship of some negative events and psychological factors to periodontal disease in an adult Swedish population 50 to 80 years of age', *Journal of Clinical Periodontology*, 29 (2002), 247–253

International Diabetes Federation, 'Facts and figures' (IDF, 2021), https://idf.org/about-diabetes/diabetes-facts-figures, accessed 7 July 2024

Michalowicz, BS et al, 'Evidence of a substantial genetic basis for risk of adult periodontitis', *Journal of Clinical Periodontology*, 71 (2000), 1699–1707

Raindi, D, 'Nutrition and periodontal disease', *Dental Update*, 43/1 (2016), 66-8

Ramseier, CA et al, 'Impact of risk factor control interventions for smoking cessation and promotion of healthy lifestyles in patients with periodontitis: A systematic review', *Journal of Clinical Periodontology*, 47 (2020), S22(90–106)

Ryder, MI et al, 'Alterations of neutrophil oxidative burst by in vitro smoke exposure: implications for oral and systemic disease', *Annals of Periodontology*, 3 (1998), 76–97

Simpson, TC et al, 'Treatment of periodontal disease for glycaemic control in people with diabetes', *Cochrane Database of Systematic Reviews*, 5 (2010), CD004714

Tomar, SL and Asma, S, 'Smoking-attributable periodontitis in the United States: Findings from NHANES III. National Health and Nutrition Examination Survey', *Journal of Periodontology*, 71 (2000), 743–751

Van Dyke, TE and Dave, S, 'Risk factors for periodontitis', *Journal of the International Academy of Periodontology*, 7/1 (2005), 3–7

Wimmer, G, Janda, M, Wieselmann-Penkner, K, Jakse, N, Polansky, R, and Pertl, C, 'Coping with stress: Its influence on periodontal disease', *Journal of Periodontology*, 73 (2002), 1343–1351

Woelber, JP et al, 'An oral health optimised diet can reduce gingival and periodontal inflammation in humans: A randomised controlled pilot study', *BMC Oral Health*, 17 (2017), 28

Zoheir, N and Hughes, FJ, 'The management of drug-influenced gingival enlargement', *Primary Dental Journal*, 8/4 (2020), 34–39

Clinical Examination

Ainamo, J and Bay, I, 'Problems and proposals for recording gingivitis and plaque', *International Dental Journal*, 25/4 (1975), 229–35

BSP, 'BPE guidelines' (BSP, 2019), www.bsperio.org.uk/assets/downloads/BSP_BPE_Guidelines_2019.pdf, accessed June 2024

Hamp, SE et al, 'Periodontal treatment of multirooted teeth: Results after 5 years', *Journal of Clinical Periodontology*, 2/3 (1975), 126–35

Miller, SC, *Textbook of Periodontia* (Blakiston Co, 1950)

O'Leary et al, 'The plaque control record', *Journal of Periodontology*, 43/1 (1972), 38

Diagnosis

Berglundh, T et al, 'Peri-implant diseases and conditions: Consensus report of workgroup 4 of the 2017 World Workshop on the Classification of Periodontal and Peri-Implant Diseases and Conditions', *Journal of Clinical Periodontology*, 45/Suppl 20 (2018), S286–S291

Caton, JG et al, 'A new classification scheme for periodontal and peri-implant diseases and conditions: Introduction and key changes from the 1999 classification', *Journal of Clinical Periodontology*, 45/Suppl 20 (2018), S1–S8

Chapple, ILC et al, 'Periodontal health and gingival diseases and conditions on an intact and a reduced periodontium. Consensus report of workgroup 1 of the 2017 World Workshop on the Classification of Periodontal and Peri-Implant Diseases and Conditions', *Journal of Clinical Periodontology*, 45/Suppl 20 (2018), S68–77

Dietrich, T et al, 'Periodontal diagnosis in the context of the 2017 classification system of periodontal diseases and conditions: Implementation in clinical practice', *British Dental Journal*, 226/1 (2019), 16–22

Jepsen, S et al, 'Periodontal manifestations of systemic diseases and developmental and acquired conditions: Consensus report of workgroup 3 of the 2017 World Workshop on the Classification of Periodontal and Peri-Implant Diseases and Conditions', *Journal of Clinical Periodontology*, 45/Suppl 20 (2018), S219–S229

Papapanou, PN et al, 'Periodontitis: Consensus report of workgroup 2 of the 2017 World Workshop on the Classification of Periodontal and Peri-Implant Diseases and Conditions', *Journal of Clinical Periodontology*, 45/Suppl 20 (2018), S162–S170

Prognosis

Mordohai, N et al, 'Factors that affect individual tooth prognosis and choices in contemporary treatment planning', *British Dental Journal*, 202/2 (2007), 63–72

Nibali, L et al, 'A retrospective study on periodontal disease progression in private practice', *Journal of Clinical Periodontology*, 44/3 (2016), 290–297

Treatment Planning

BSP, 'BSP guidelines for patient referral' (BSP, 2020), www.bsperio.org.uk/assets/downloads/BSP_Guidelines_for_Patient_Referral_2020.pdf, accessed June 2024

Herrera, D et al, 'Treatment of stage IV periodontitis: The EFP S3 level clinical practice guideline', *Journal of Clinical Periodontology*, 49/S24 (2022), 4–71

Sanz, M et al, 'Treatment of stage I–III periodontitis: The EFP S3 level clinical practice guideline', *Journal of Clinical Periodontology*, 47/S22 (2020), 4–60

West, N et al, 'BSP implementation of European S3-level evidence-based treatment guidelines for stage I–III periodontitis in UK clinical practice', *Journal of Dentistry*, 106 (2021), 103562

Educating And Empowering Patients

Michie, S, Van Stralen, MM, and West, R, 'The behaviour change wheel: A new method for characterising and designing behaviour change interventions', *Implementation Science*, 6/1 (2011), 1–12

Sanz, M et al, 'Treatment of stage I–III periodontitis: The EFP S3 level clinical practice guideline', *Journal of Clinical Periodontology*, 47/S22 (2020), 4–60

Scottish Dental Effectiveness Programme – Oral Hygiene TIPPS (SDCEP), www.periodontalcare.sdcep.org.uk/supporting-tools/oral-hygiene-tipps, accessed 27 July 2024

Slot, DE, Valkenburg, C, and Van der Weijden, F, 'Mechanical plaque removal of periodontal maintenance patients: A systematic review and network meta-analysis', *Journal of Clinical Periodontology*, 47/Suppl 22 (2020), 107–124

Tonetti, MS et al, 'Principles in prevention of periodontal diseases: Consensus report of group 1 of the 11th European Workshop on Periodontology on effective prevention of periodontal and peri-implant diseases', *Journal of Clinical Periodontology*, 42/S16 (2015), S5–11

Yaacob, M et al, 'Powered versus manual toothbrushing for oral health', *Cochrane Database of Systematic Reviews*, 6 (2014), CD002281

Non-Surgical Periodontal Therapy

Badersten, A et al, 'Effect of nonsurgical periodontal therapy. I. Moderately advanced periodontitis', *Journal of Clinical Periodontology*, 8 (1981), 57–72

Cobb, CM, 'Non-surgical pocket therapy: Mechanical', *Annals of Periodontology*, 1 (1996), 443–490

Da Costa, LFNP et al, 'Chlorhexidine mouthwash as an adjunct to mechanical therapy in chronic periodontitis: A meta-analysis', *Journal of the American Dental Association*, 148/5 (2017), 308–318

Drisko, CH, 'Root instrumentation: Power-driven versus manual scalers, which one?', *Dental Clinics of North America*, 42 (1998), 229–244

Graziani, F et al, 'Acute-phase response following full-mouth versus quadrant non-surgical periodontal treatment: A randomised clinical trial', *Journal of Clinical Periodontology*, 42/9 (2015), 843–852

Graziani, F et al, 'Acute-phase response following one-stage full-mouth versus quadrant non-surgical periodontal treatment in subjects with comorbid type 2 diabetes: A randomised clinical trial', *Journal of Clinical Periodontology*, 50/4 (2023), 487–499

Herrera, D et al, 'Adjunctive effect of locally delivered antimicrobials in periodontitis therapy: A systematic review and meta-analysis', *Journal of Clinical Periodontology*, 47 (2020), 239–256

Loos, B et al, 'An evaluation of basic periodontal therapy using sonic and ultrasonic scaler', *Journal of Clinical Periodontology*, 14 (1987) 29–33

Mehta, J et al, 'Minimally invasive non-surgical periodontal therapy of intrabony defects: A prospective multi-centre cohort study', *Journal of Clinical Periodontology*, 51/7 (2024), 905–914

Nibali, L et al, 'Minimally invasive non-surgical vs surgical approach for periodontal intrabony defects: A randomised controlled trial', *Trials*, 20/1 (2019), 461

Sanz, M et al, 'Treatment of stage I–III periodontitis: The EFP S3 level clinical practice guideline', *Journal of Clinical Periodontology*, 47/S22 (2020), 4–60

Suvan, J et al, 'Subgingival instrumentation for treatment of periodontitis: A systematic review', *Journal of Clinical Periodontology*, 47/Suppl 22 (2020), 155–175

Tomasi, C et al, 'A randomised multi-centre study on the effectiveness of non-surgical periodontal therapy in general practice', *Journal of Clinical Periodontology*, 49/11 (2022), 1092–1105

Periodontal Challenges

Occlusal trauma and splinting

Cortellini, P et al, 'The simplified papilla preservation flap in the regenerative treatment of deep intrabony defects: Clinical outcomes and postoperative morbidity', *Journal of Periodontology*, 72/12 (2001), 1702–1712

Fan, J and Caton, JG, 'Occlusal trauma and excessive occlusal forces: Narrative review, case definitions and diagnostic considerations', *Journal of Periodontology*, 89/S1 (2018), S214–S222

Ferencz, J, 'Splinting', *Dental Clinics of North America*, 313 (1987), 383–393

Hirschfield, I, 'The individual missing tooth: A factor in dental and periodontal disease', *Journal of the American Dental Association*, 24 (1937), 67–82

Jepsen, S et al, 'Periodontal manifestations of systemic diseases and developmental and acquired conditions: Consensus report of workgroup 3 of the 2017 World Workshop on the Classification of Periodontal and Peri-Implant Diseases and Conditions', *Journal of Clinical Periodontology*, 45/Suppl 20 (2018), S219–S229

Nyman, SR and Lang, NP, 'Tooth mobility and the biologic rationale for splinting teeth', *Periodontology 2000*, 4 (1994), 15–22

Passanezi, E and Sant'Ana, ACP, 'Role of occlusion in periodontal disease', *Periodontology 2000*, 79 (2019), 129–150

Furcations

American Academy of Periodontology, Glossary of Periodontal Terms, 4th edition (American Academy of Periodontology, 2001), https://members.perio.org/libraries/glossary, accessed 1 August 2024

Hughes, FJ, *Clinical Problem Solving in Periodontology and Implantology*, 1st edition (Churchill Livingstone Elsevier, 2013)

Jepsen, S et al, 'Regenerative surgical treatment of furcation defects: A systematic review and Bayesian network meta-analysis of randomised clinical trials', *Journal of Clinical Periodontology*, 47/S22 (2020), 352–374

Dentine hypersensitivity

Holland, GR et al, 'Guidelines for the design and conduct of clinical trials on dentine hypersensitivity', *Journal of Clinical Periodontology*, 24 (1997), 808–813

West, NX et al, 'Prevalence of dentine hypersensitivity and study of associated factors: A European population-based cross-sectional study', *Journal of Dentistry*, 41 (2013), 841–851

West, N et al, 'Management of dentine hypersensitivity: Efficacy of professionally and self-administered agents', *Journal of Clinical Periodontology*, 42/S16 (2015), S256–S302.

Halitosis

Eli, I et al, 'Attribution of bad breath to halitosis and its impact on social interactions', *Journal of Dental Research*, 80/8 (2001), 2083–2086

Friedman, M et al, 'Management of halitosis', *Dental Clinics of North America*, 59/1 (2015), 159–178

Greenman, J et al, 'The science of bad breath: Overview of causes and treatments', *Journal of Dental Research*, 84/7 (2005), 606–614

Kumar, P et al, 'Halitosis: A review', *International Journal of Oral Health Sciences*, 4/1 (2014), 22–26

Miller, D and Dyer, J, 'Halitosis: An overview', *Dental Clinics of North America*, 55/4 (2011), 771–782

Outhouse, TL et al, 'Tongue scraping for treating halitosis', *Cochrane Database of Systematic Reviews*, 19/2 (2006), CD005519

Roldán, S et al, 'The role of tongue coating in halitosis', *BMC Oral Health*, 13 (2013), 23

Rosenberg, M et al, 'Halitosis: A review of the literature', *Journal of Clinical Dentistry*, 17/1 (2006), 8-12

Sanz, M et al, 'Effect of professional mechanical plaque removal on secondary prevention of periodontitis and the complications of gingival and periodontal preventive measures: Consensus report of group 4 of the 11th European workshop on periodontology on effective prevention of periodontal and peri-implant diseases', *Journal of Clinical Periodontology*, 42/Suppl 16 (2015), S214–S220

Scully, C et al, 'Halitosis (bad breath): A review', *Oral Diseases*, 7/6 (2001), 230–233

Slot, DE et al, 'Management of oral mal-odour. Efficacy of mechanical and/or chemical agents: A systematic review', *Journal of Clinical Periodontology*, 42/16 (2015), S303–16

Van Dorsten, FA and Van der Weijden, GA, 'Prevalence of halitosis: A review of the literature', *Journal of Clinical Periodontology*, 34/6 (2007), 415–422

Yoshida, Y et al, 'Clinical evaluation of halitosis: An organoleptic approach', *Journal of Oral Rehabilitation*, 41/1 (2014), 70–76

Periodontal Emergencies And Their

American Academy of Periodontology, 'Parameter on acute periodontal diseases, parameters of care (supplement)', *Journal of Periodontology*, 71 (2000), 863–866

Creath, CJ et al, 'A case report: Gingival swelling due to a fingernail-biting habit', *Journal of the American Dental Association*, 126 (1995), 1019–1021

De Bruyne, MA et al, 'Necrosis of the gingiva caused by calcium hydroxide: A case report', International Endodontic Journal, 33 (2000), 67–71

Dello Russo, NM, 'The post-prophylaxis periodontal abscess: Etiology and treatment', *International Journal of Periodontics & Restorative Dentistry*, 1985; 5 (1985), 28–37

Fine, DH, 'Microbial identification and antibiotic sensitivity testing, an aid for patients refractory to periodontal therapy: A report of 3 cases', *Journal of Clinical Periodontology*, 21 (1994), 98–106

Garrett, S et al, 'Comparison of a bioabsorbable GTR barrier to a non-absorbable barrier in treating human class II furcation defects. A multi-center parallel design randomised single-blind trial', *Journal of Periodontology*, 68 (1997), 667–675

Gillette, WB and Van House, RL, 'Ill effects of improper oral hygiene procedure', *Journal of the American Dentistry Association*, 101 (1980), 476

Helovuo, H et al, 'Changes in the prevalence of subgingival enteric rods, staphylococci and yeasts after treatment with penicillin and erythromycin', *Oral Microbiology and Immunology*, 8 (1993), 75–79

Herrera, D et al, 'The periodontal abscess (I): Clinical and microbiological findings', *Journal of Clinical Periodontology*, 27 (2000), 387–394

Herrera, D et al, 'Acute periodontal lesions', *Periodontology 2000*, 65 (2014), 149–177

Krejci, CB, 'Self-inflicted gingival injury due to habitual fingernail biting', *Journal of Periodontology*, 71 (2000), 1029–1031

Loesche, WJ et al, 'The bacteriology of acute necrotising ulcerative gingivitis', *Journal of Periodontology*, 53 (1982), 223–30

Sapir, S and Bimstein, E, 'Cholinsalicylate gel induced oral lesion: Report of case', *Journal of Clinical Paediatric Dentistry*, 24 (2000), 103–106

Supportive Periodontal Care

Cortellini, P and Tonetti, MS, 'Periodontal risk assessment in clinical practice: A review', *International Journal of Periodontics and Restorative Dentistry*, 25/4 (2005), 397–404

Genco, R et al, 'Relationship of stress, distress, and inadequate coping behaviors to periodontal disease', *Journal of Periodontology*, 70/7 (1999), 711–723

Heasman, L et al, 'The effect of smoking on periodontal treatment response: A review of clinical evidence', *Journal of Clinical Periodontology*, 33/4 (2006): 241–253

Kornman, KS et al, 'The interleukin-1 genotype as a severity factor in adult periodontal disease', *Journal of Clinical Periodontology*, 24/1 (1997), 72–77

Löe, H, 'Periodontal disease: The sixth complication of diabetes mellitus', *Diabetes Care*, 16/1 (1993), 329–334

Mavridis, I and Mavridis, K, 'The significance of tooth type and periodontal maintenance in the prognosis of multi-rooted teeth', *Journal of Periodontology*, 89/11 (2018), 1346–1355

Meyer, DH and Lewis, RA, 'Assessing periodontal disease risk: An evaluation of the DEPPA tool', *Journal of Periodontal Research*, 53/5 (2018), 683–689

Rosling, B et al, 'Longitudinal periodontal tissue alterations during supportive therapy', *Journal of Clinical Periodontology*, 28 (2001), 241–249

Tomar, SL and Asma, S, 'Smoking-attributable periodontitis in the United States: Findings from NHANES III', *Journal of Periodontology*, 7/5 (2000), 743–751

Trombelli, L et al, 'The role of bleeding on probing in periodontal diagnosis: A systematic review', *Journal of Periodontology*, 86/6 (2015), 665–676

Dental Implants

Brånemark, PI et al, 'Osseointegration and its clinical significance', *Journal of Oral Rehabilitation*, 4/4 (1977), 277-291

Feine, JS et al, 'The McGill consensus statement on overdentures recommends mandibular two-implant overdentures choice standard of care for edentulous patients', *Gerodontology*, 19/1 (2002), 3-4

Friedman, N et al, 'Interventions for the management of peri-implantitis', *Cochrane Database of Systematic Reviews*, 12 (2012), CD008811

Herrera, D et al, 'Treatment of stage IV periodontitis: The EFP S3 level clinical practice guideline', *Journal of Clinical Periodontology*, 49/S24 (2022), 4-71

Jung, RE and Ganeles, J, 'Periodontal and peri-implant tissues: Differences in anatomy and physiology', *Periodontology 2000*, 63/1 (2013), 101-112

Kumar, S et al, 'Comparative analysis of the longevity of retained natural teeth versus dental implants', *International Journal of Prosthodontics*, 28/3 (2015), 287-292

Lang, NP et al, 'Peri-implantitis: A complication of dental implants in patients with periodontitis', *Periodontology 2000*, 55/1 (2011), 47-56

Misch, CE et al, 'The importance of preserving teeth in patients with periodontal disease', *Dental Clinics of North America*, 58/3 (2014), 437-454

Nishihara, Y et al, 'Comparative histological study of peri-implant and periodontal tissues', *Journal of Periodontology*, 86/4 (2015), 508-516

Pjetursson, BE and Lang, NP, 'Comparative survival and complication rates of tooth-supported fixed dental prostheses and implant-supported fixed dental prostheses', *Clinical Oral Implants Research*, 19/2 (2008), 97-109

Pjetursson, BE et al, 'Peri-implantitis susceptibility as it relates to periodontal therapy and supportive care', *Clinical Oral Implants Research*, 23/7 (2012), 888–94

Roccuzzo, A et al, 'Longitudinal assessment of peri-implant diseases in patients with and without history of periodontitis: A 20-year follow-up study', *International Journal of Oral Implantology*, 16/3 (2023), 211–222

Salgado, JM et al, 'Influence of cement excess on the development of peri-implant diseases: A review', *International Journal of Oral & Maxillofacial Implants*, 31/3 (2016), 594–599

Sanz, M et al, 'Periodontal and peri-implant diseases: A comprehensive review', *Journal of Clinical Periodontology*, 42/ S16 (2015), S30–S50

Schwarz, F et al, 'Peri-implant diseases: A review of the literature', *International Journal of Oral & Maxillofacial Implants*, 26/5 (2011), 110–118

Schwarz, F et al, 'The influence of inter-implant distance on the long-term success of dental implants', *Clinical Oral Implants Research*, 26/6 (2015), 692–699

Sgolastra, F et al, 'Periodontitis, implant loss and peri-implantitis. A meta-analysis', *Clinical Oral Implants Research*, 26/4 (2015), e8–e16

Zitzmann, NU and Marinello, CP, 'Patient satisfaction with implant-supported overdentures compared with conventional dentures', *International Journal of Prosthodontics*, 14/6 (2001), 596–602

Multidisciplinary Care

The perio–endo interface

Friedman, S and Stabholtz, A, 'Endodontic and periodontal interrelationships', *Endodontic Topics*, 3/1 (1999), 87–97

Kumar, P, and Nisha K, 'Endodontic-periodontic interrelationship: A review', *Journal of Clinical and Diagnostic Research*, 9/2 (2015), ZE01–ZE05

Papapanou, PN et al, 'Periodontitis: Consensus report of workgroup 2 of the 2017 World Workshop on the Classification of Periodontal and Peri-Implant Diseases and Conditions', *Journal of Clinical Periodontology*, 45/Suppl 20 (2018), S162–S170

Santos, JC et al, 'The association between endodontic and periodontal lesions: A review', *Journal of Clinical Periodontology*, 44/11 (2017), 1064–1072

The perio–ortho interface

Bishara, SE et al, 'Relapse in orthodontics: A review of the literature', *American Journal of Orthodontics and Dentofacial Orthopedics*, 154/2 (2018), 184–193

Diem, V et al, 'The role of temporary anchorage devices in orthodontics for periodontally compromised patients', *European Journal of Orthodontics*, 41/3 (2019), 304–311

García, J et al, 'Gingival overgrowth in orthodontics: A review', *European Journal of Orthodontics*, 42/5 (2020), 509–515

Hassan, M et al, 'Monitoring periodontal health during orthodontic therapy', *American Journal of Orthodontics and Dentofacial Orthopedics*, 156/5 (2019), 685–691

Herrera, D et al, 'Treatment of stage IV periodontitis: The EFP S3 level clinical practice guideline', *Journal of Clinical Periodontology*, 49/S24 (2022), 4–71

Keller, M et al, 'The impact of orthodontic treatment on periodontal health: A systematic review', *Orthodontics & Craniofacial Research*, 24/3 (2021), 180–192

Kloukos, D et al, 'Effect of combined periodontal and orthodontic treatment of tilted molars and of teeth with intrabony and furcation defects in stage-IV periodontitis patients: A systematic review', *Journal of Clinical Periodontology*, 49/Suppl 24 (2021), S121–S148

Kothiwale, S et al, 'Orthodontic considerations in patients with periodontal disease: A review', *Journal of Indian Orthodontic Society*, 54/1 (2020), 24–31

Kumar, P et al, 'Oral hygiene and periodontal management during orthodontic treatment', *Journal of Clinical Orthodontics*, 54/6 (2020a), 365–372

Kumar, P et al, 'Lifelong retention protocols in orthodontics: A clinical perspective', *Journal of Clinical Orthodontics*, 54/5 (2020b), 273–279

Lindhe, J et al, 'Periodontal health and orthodontics: Considerations for tooth movement in patients with periodontitis', *Periodontology 2000*, 68/1 (2015), 187–203

Martin, C et al, 'Effect of orthodontic therapy in periodontitis and non-periodontitis patients: A systematic review with meta-analysis', *Journal of Clinical Periodontology*, 49/Suppl 24 (2021), S72–S101

Mason, A et al, 'Efficacy of different retention strategies after orthodontic treatment: A systematic review', *European Journal of Orthodontics*, 41/3 (2019), 238–247

Miller, D et al, 'Clear aligners vs traditional braces: A review of the literature', *Journal of Clinical Orthodontics*, 55/5 (2021), 283–290

O'Leary, C et al, 'Understanding the cone effect in orthodontics', *The Angle Orthodontist*, 91/1 (2021), 27–32

Papageorgiou, SN et al, 'Effect of periodontal-orthodontic treatment of teeth with pathological tooth flaring, drifting and elongation in patients with severe periodontitis: A systematic review with meta-analysis', *Journal of Clinical Periodontology*, 49/Suppl 24 (2021), S102–S120

Sanz, M et al, 'Treatment of stage I–III periodontitis: The EFP S3 level clinical practice guideline', *Journal of Clinical Periodontology*, 47/S22 (2020), 4–60

Watanabe, H et al, 'Orthodontic treatment for patients with periodontitis: a systematic review', *American Journal of Orthodontics and Dentofacial Orthopedics*, 157/1 (2020), 17–25

Pocket Reduction Surgery

Aapeng, F et al, 'Factors influencing the healing of periodontal tissues after surgical treatment', *International Journal of Oral Science*, 15/1 (2023), 10–19

Aroca, E and Mombelli, A, 'Periodontal regeneration: The role of mobility', *Periodontology 2000*, 68/1 (2015), 46–56

Bartlett, JD, 'Amelogenins: Structure, function and role in tooth development', *Nature Reviews: Molecular Cell Biology*, 14/12 (2013), 829–844

Bichara, DA et al, 'The role of enamel matrix proteins in wound healing', *Journal of Tissue Engineering*, 8 (2017), 2041731417710421

Buser, D et al, 'Guided bone regeneration with Bio-Gide and bone grafts in the maxilla', *International Journal of Oral & Maxillofacial Implants*, 30/3 (2015), 505–512

Caffesse, RG et al, 'A comparison of non-surgical and surgical periodontal therapy', *Journal of Periodontology*, 57/4 (1986), 232–238

Cobb, CM, 'Non-surgical pocket therapy: A review of the literature', *Journal of Periodontology*, 67/9 (1996), 933–949

Cortellini, P et al, 'Long-term outcomes of surgical periodontal therapy: A systematic review', *Periodontology 2000*, 75/1 (2017), 70–80

Cortellini, P and Tonetti, MS, 'A minimally invasive surgical approach to the management of intra-bony defects', *Journal of Clinical Periodontology*, 32/S6 (2005), 190–196

Friedman, N, 'A technique for periodontal surgery', *Journal of Periodontology*, 33/1 (1962), 66–72

Garg, V, Ranjan, R, and Ranjan, R, 'The role of non-surgical periodontal therapy in treating periodontitis: A review', *Journal of Periodontology*, 93/5 (2022), 633–642

Greenstein, G and Cavallaro, J, 'Surgical and nonsurgical treatment of furcation involvement: A review', *International Journal of Periodontics & Restorative Dentistry*, 26/5 (2006), 455–461

Haffajee, AD and Socransky, SS, 'The effect of periodontal therapy on the microbiological composition of subgingival plaque', *Journal of Clinical Periodontology*, 21/1 (1994), 33–41

Hämmerle, CHF and Trombelli, L, 'Guided bone regeneration in implant dentistry', *Periodontology 2000*, 73/1 (2017), 145–157

Huang, TH et al, 'Minimally invasive techniques in periodontal surgery: A review', *Journal of Dental Sciences*, 12/2 (2017), 107–114

Karnik, A et al, 'The importance of the role of gingival contours in periodontal therapy', *Journal of Clinical Dentistry*, 10/1 (1999), 29–34

Kirkland, L, 'A method of periodontal surgery', *The Dental Review*, 58/6 (1931), 505–510

Lindhe, J et al, 'Critical probing depths in periodontal therapy', *Journal of Clinical Periodontology*, 9/4 (1982), 323–36

Löe, H, 'Periodontal disease: The sixth complication of diabetes mellitus', *Diabetes Care*, 11/3 (1988), 275–276

McGuire, MK and Nunn, ME, 'Prognosis versus actual treatment outcomes', *International Journal of Periodontics and Restorative Dentistry*, 16/1 (1996), 1–11

Müller, HP and Heine, S, 'Critical probing depth: An important concept in periodontal therapy', *Clinical Oral Investigations*, 23/4 (2019), 1797–1806

Nanci, A et al, 'The role of enamel matrix derivative in periodontal regeneration', *Periodontology 2000*, 81/1 (2019), 185–202

Neumann, M, 'Die operativen Möglichkeiten in der Parodontaltherapie', *Dtsch Zahnarztl Z*, 22 (1920), 1013–1018

Nibali, L et al, 'Surgical and non-surgical management of intra-bony defects: A systematic review', *Journal of Clinical Periodontology*, 46/1 (2019), 29–44

Nyman, S et al, 'Periodontal surgery in plaque-infected dentitions', *Journal of Clinical Periodontology*, 4/4 (1977), 240–9

Nyman, S et al, 'Healing of human periodontal tissues after treatment', *Journal of Clinical Periodontology*, 9/4 (1982), 259–271

Ramfjord, SP and Nissle, RR, 'The modified Widman flap', *Journal of Periodontology*, 45/10 (1974), 613–617

Sanz, M et al, 'Treatment of stage I–III periodontitis: The EFP S3 level clinical practice guideline', *Journal of Clinical Periodontology*, 47/S22 (2020), 4–60

Scabbia, A et al, 'Cigarette smoking negatively affects healing response following flap debridement surgery', *Journal of Periodontology*, 72/1 (2001), 43–9

Schlegel, K et al, 'Bone regeneration in dental applications: Biological effects of Bio-Oss', *Clinical Oral Implants Research*, 26/4 (2015), 424–430

Sgolastra, F et al, 'Minimally invasive surgery in periodontology: A systematic review', *Journal of Clinical Periodontology*, 43/4 (2016), 282–293

Socransky, SS et al, 'The role of the microbiota in the pathogenesis of periodontal disease', *Journal of Clinical Periodontology*, 11/4 (1984), 168–178

Stern, R et al, 'Enamel matrix derivative in the treatment of periodontal defects', *Journal of Clinical Periodontology*, 36/1 (2009), 12–21

Tornes, K et al, 'Smoking and the treatment of periodontitis: A review of the literature', *Journal of Periodontology*, 76/11 (2005), 2050–2057

Trombelli, L et al, 'Surgical treatment of intrabony defects: A systematic review', *Journal of Clinical Periodontology*, 40/1 (2013), 1–15

Trombelli, L et al, 'Periodontal regeneration: A critical review of the literature', *Periodontology 2000*, 66/1 (2014), 153–171

Vignoletti, F and Sanz, M, 'Influence of endodontic status on the outcomes of regenerative periodontal therapy', *Journal of Clinical Periodontology*, 41/9 (2014), 913–920

Wagner, W and Gmür, R, 'The critical probing depth in predicting the outcome of non-surgical and surgical periodontal therapy', *Journal of Clinical Periodontology*, 20/7 (1993), 431–434

Widman, G, 'Über die Entfernung des Zahnhalteapparates', *Dtsch Zahnarztl Z*, 22 (1918)

Yamada, Y et al, 'Impact of papilla preservation flaps on periodontal regeneration: A systematic review', *Journal of Clinical Periodontology*, 47/9 (2020), 1037–1049

Gingival Recession And Surgery

Allen, A, 'Use of the supraperiosteal envelope in soft tissue grafting for root coverage. II. Clinical results', *International Journal of Periodontics and Restorative Dentistry*, 14 (1994), 302–315

Baker, SR et al, 'Periodontal phenotypes: What do we know and what do we need to know?', *Journal of Clinical Periodontology*, 45/5 (2018), 498–507

Baldi, C et al, 'Coronally advanced flap procedure for root coverage. Is flap thickness a relevant predictor to achieve root coverage? A 19-case series', *Journal of Periodontology*, 70 (1999), 1077–1084

Cairo, F et al, 'Aesthetic surgical correction of gingival recession: Case reports and scientific evidence', *Journal of Esthetic and Restorative Dentistry*, 30/4 (2018), 332–340

Cortellini, P and Bissada, NF, 'Mucogingival conditions in the natural dentition: Narrative review, case definitions, and diagnostic considerations', *Journal of Periodontology*, 89/S1 (2018), S204–S213

Jepsen, S et al, 'Periodontal manifestations of systemic diseases and developmental and acquired conditions: consensus report of workgroup 3 of the 2017 World Workshop on the Classification of Periodontal and Peri-Implant Diseases and Conditions', *Journal of Clinical Periodontology*, 45/Suppl 20 (2018), S219–S229

Khan, S et al, 'Gingival recession: Its causes and management', *International Journal of Health Sciences*, 10/1 (2016), 265–278

Miller, PD, 'A classification of marginal tissue recession', *International Journal of Periodontics and Restorative Dentistry*, 5 (1985), 8–13

Tinti, C et al, 'Guided tissue regeneration in the treatment of human facial recession: A 12-case report', *Journal of Periodontology*, 64/3 (1992), 119–124

Tonetti, MS and Jepsen, S, 'Clinical efficacy of periodontal plastic surgery procedures: Consensus report of Group 2 of the 10th European Workshop on Periodontology', *Journal of Clinical Periodontology*, 41/S15 (2014), S36–S43

Trombelli, L, 'Periodontal regeneration in deep intrabony defects: A systematic review', *Journal of Clinical Periodontology*, 42/S16 (2015), S116–S132

Zhang, Y et al, 'Impact of oral hygiene on the success of periodontal plastic surgery: A systematic review', *Journal of Periodontology*, 92/4 (2021), 436–446

Zucchelli, G and De Sanctis, M, 'Treatment of multiple recession-type defects in patients with aesthetic demands', *Journal of Periodontology*, 71/9 (2000), 1506–1514

Crown-Lengthening Surgery

Cairo, F et al, 'Aesthetic surgical correction of gingival recession: Case reports and scientific evidence', *Journal of Esthetic and Restorative Dentistry*, 30/4 (2018), 332–340

Chu, SJ et al, 'Aesthetic parameters for gingival zenith position: A review of the literature', *Journal of Esthetic and Restorative Dentistry*, 21/6 (2009), 373–384

Cohen, ES, *Atlas of Cosmetic & Reconstructive Periodontal Surgery*, Vol 3 (Hamilton, 2007)

Cortellini, P and Bissada, NF, 'Mucogingival conditions in the natural dentition: Narrative review, case definitions, and diagnostic considerations', *Journal of Periodontology*, 89/S1 (2018), S204–S213

Coslet, GJ, Vanarsdall, R, and Weisgold, A, 'Diagnosis and classification of delayed passive eruption of the dentogingival junction in the adult', *Alpha Omegan*, 10 (1977), 24–8

Garber, DA and Salama, MA, 'The aesthetic smile: Diagnosis and treatment', *Periodontology 2000*, 11/1 (1996), 18–28

Garguilo, AW, Wentz, FM, and Orban, B, 'Dimensions and relations of the dentogingival junction in humans', *Journal of Periodontology*, 32 (1961), 321

Gargiulo, AW et al, 'The importance of tooth proportion in the aesthetics of the smile', *Journal of Esthetic and Restorative Dentistry*, 18/1 (2006), 43–52

Goldman, HM and Cohen, DW, 'The effect of altered passive eruption on periodontal health', *Journal of Periodontology*, 42/1 (1971), 28–32

Jepsen, S et al, 'Periodontal manifestations of systemic diseases and developmental and acquired conditions: consensus report of workgroup 3 of the 2017 World Workshop on the Classification of Periodontal and Peri-Implant Diseases and Conditions', *Journal of Clinical Periodontology*, 45/Suppl 20 (2018), S219–S229

The Author

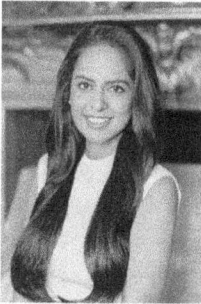

Dr Reena Wadia is the founder and principal periodontist at RW Perio, which she set up and grew into an established, state-of-the-art, four-clinic surgery on Harley Street. Today, RW Perio is one of the top specialist periodontal clinics in the UK.

Dr Reena's mission is to highlight the importance of gum health, incorporating it into a healthy overall lifestyle. This focus has been celebrated regularly in the press, including *Forbes, Financial Times How To Spend It, Vogue, Harper's Bazaar, The Times,* and the BBC. She has developed her own award-winning product range, By Dr Reena, which combines specialist dentistry with luxury lifestyle. Her podcast, *Life & Smile,* was launched in 2022, featuring guests including Sarah Harris (*British Vogue*), Lydia Slater (*Harper's Bazaar*), and Harpz Kaur (BBC).

As well as being passionate about acquiring new knowledge, Dr Reena has always encouraged and supported other entrepreneurs, dentists, and hygienists/therapists by sharing her own learning and experiences. She is the founder of Perio School, which is now the leading global teaching academy for periodontal courses, having taught dental students, dentists, and hygienists for over ten years.

Dr Reena endeavours to contribute to the profession through her role as an expert advisor on the BDA Indemnity Board, as co-editor of the 'Other Journals in Brief' section of the *British Dental Journal*, and as trustee of the Oral and Dental Research Trust.

- ⊕ www.perio.school
- ⊕ www.rwperio.com
- ⊕ www.bydrreena.com
- in www.linkedin.com/in/reenawadia
- ⊙ @reenawadia
- ▶ www.youtube.com/rwperio

www.ingramcontent.com/pod-product-compliance
Lightning Source LLC
Chambersburg PA
CBHW061147220326
41599CB00025B/4379